Neuro-Ophthalmology and Orbital Disease

Diagnosis and Treatment

Handbook of
Neuro-Ophthalmology and Orbital Disease
Diagnosis and Treatment
SECOND EDITION

ROBERT L. TOMSAK, MD, PhD
Associate Professor, Department of Neurology
and Ophthalmology
Case Western Reserve University School of Medicine;
Director, Division of Clinical Neuro-Ophthalmology
Department of Neurology, University Hospitals of Cleveland
Cleveland, Ohio

MARK R. LEVINE, MD, FACS
Clinical Professor, Department of Ophthalmology
Case Western Reserve University School of Medicine;
Head, Oculoplastic Section, Department of Ophthalmology
University Hospitals of Cleveland
Cleveland, Ohio

BUTTERWORTH
HEINEMANN
An Imprint of Elsevier

BUTTERWORTH
HEINEMANN

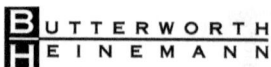

An imprint of Elsevier

The Curtis Center
Independence Square West
Philadelphia, Pennsylvania 19106

HANDBOOK OF NEURO-OPHTHALMOLOGY AND   0-7506-7417-2
ORBITAL DISEASE: DIAGNOSIS AND TREATMENT, Second Edition
Copyright © 2004, Elsevier (USA). All rights reserved.

NOTICE

Neuro-ophthalmology is an ever-changing field. Standard safety precautions must be followed, but as new research and clinical experience broaden our knowledge, changes in treatment and drug therapy may become necessary or appropriate. Readers are advised to check the most current product information provided by the manufacturer of each drug to be administered to verify the recommended dose, the method and duration of administration, and contraindications. It is the responsibility of the treating physician, relying on experience and knowledge of the patient, to determine dosages and the best treatment for each individual patient. Neither the publisher nor the author assumes any liability for any injury and/or damage to persons or property arising from this publication.

Previous edition copyrighted 1997

International Standard Book Number 0-7506-7417-2

Aquisitions Editor: Paul Fam
Publishing Services Manager: Patricia Tannian
Project Manager: Sarah Wunderly
Design Manager: Gail Morey Hudson
Cover Design: PrePress Imaging, Inc.

Transferred to Digital Printing in 2009

In memory of
Jonathan Robert Tomsak
Requiescat in peace
August 18, 2002

Acknowledgment
Thanks to my office staff
Pat Podbielski and **Dawn Weiss**
for all their help in taking care of our patients

Preface to the Second Edition

In this edition of *Handbook of Neuro-Ophthalmology and Orbital Disease*, the original 17 chapters from the first edition have been updated and five new chapters covering aspects of orbital disease have been written by Dr. Mark Levine. Mark is an exceptional oculoplastic surgeon, ophthalmologist, and teacher and is also a long-time friend and colleague.

I want to thank my colleagues in neuro-ophthalmology at University Hospitals of Cleveland for their collaboration and stimulation. They include, but are not limited to, Bob Daroff, John Leigh, Lou Dell'Osso, Henry Kaminski, and Janet Rucker. Also, I continue to look back to my fellowship year (1979) with J. Lawton Smith at the Bascom Palmer Eye Institute as the best professional year of my life. More than anyone JLS taught me to be a "treatin' doctor," and I hope that this approach to neuro-ophthalmology is evident in this book.

Robert L. Tomsak
2003

Preface to the First Edition

Neuro-ophthalmology is usually thought of as a diagnostic subspecialty. Yet clinical neuro-ophthalmologists are faced with treatment issues on a daily basis. I have chosen to briefly discuss 17 topics that have significant therapeutic implications — they are the "bread and butter" of my practice. I have tried to make the discussions short and to the point, current, and scholarly.

Treatment issues in some of these areas are controversial. I have tried to present the controversies in an unbiased way, but I have not refrained from speculating at times, or from stating my opinions or personal experience.

This handbook is aimed at physicians at the resident level and up, and is produced in a size that allows transportation into the "trenches," where it is intended to be used the most. I thank Margaret Brown for photographic assistance.

I hope this book helps in the care of your patients.

Robert L. Tomsak

Contents

I

NEURO-OPHTHALMOLOGY

1

Anterior Ischemic Optic Neuropathy

OVERVIEW AND ETIOLOGY

Anterior ischemic optic neuropathy (AION) presents as sudden, painless loss of vision associated with optic disc edema and results from infarction of the optic disc in the perilaminar region [1-3]. The nonarteritic form of the disease (NAION) is most common and occurs in patients over the age of 45. Systemic diseases such as hypertension, diabetes mellitus, coronary artery disease, and hypercholesterolemia [4] often accompany NAION, but the patients are usually in functional good health. Other associations may include cigarette smoking [5], gastrointestinal ulcer, thyroid disease, chronic obstructive pulmonary disease [6], antiphospholipid antibodies, elevated plasma fibrinogen, and elevated intraocular pressure [7-9]. NAION is often noted on awakening, and nocturnal hypotension has been implicated as a cause [10], as has sleep apnea [11]. Also, unlike in arteritic ischemic optic neuropathy, there is no evidence that thrombosis of nutrient arteries to the optic nerve head is a significant precipitating factor in NAION [12]. Structural factors may also play a role in NAION because most patients have small cup-to-disc (C/D) ratios [13-15] (an appearance characterized by Burde as "the disc at risk" [16]). Fellow eye involvement happens approximately 15% of the time [17]. Patients with NAION seem to have more ischemic white matter lesions as demonstrated by magnetic resonance imaging (MRI) [18].

Differentiation of the arteritic from the nonarteritic form of AION is exceptionally important because the severity of vision loss in arteritic AION is much greater and requires prompt treatment with corticosteroids. The distinction between the two forms can usually be made by an examination of patient history and clinical features, as well as the use of abnormal acute phase reactants and positive temporal artery biopsy (see Chapter 14).

Arteritic AION (Table 1-1) occurs less frequently than NAION, occurs in an older age group (≥60 years) and is more prevalent in white females. Classic symptoms of temporal arteritis and polymyalgia rheumatica are often present.

Even less frequently, NAION occurs after cataract extraction [19], ipsilateral carotid artery occlusion [20], or open-heart surgery [21]. Embolic ischemic optic neuropathy is most unusual and deserves mention only to emphasize that an extensive evaluation for carotid artery atherosclerosis or heart valve disease is usually unwarranted in patients with isolated AION [22,23]. An exception should be made if emboli are seen in the retinal vessels or if permanent visual loss is

Table 1-1   Some Features Differentiating Arteritic from Nonarteritic Anterior Ischemic Optic Neuropathy (AION)

Feature	Arteritic AION	Nonarteritic AION
Age	≥60 yrs	≥45 yrs
Sex	More prevalent in females	No difference
Vision loss	Sudden, severe, progressive	Sudden, less severe, rarely progressive
Transient monocular blindness	Rare	Never
Bilateral involvement	Common: rapid	About 15%; months, years
Optic cup size	Normal	Small
Systemic symptoms of giant cell arteritis	Usually	None
Erythrocyte sedimentation rate and fibrinogen	Elevated	Normal

preceded by transient monocular blindness [24]. Other rare AION presentations include bilateral simultaneous AION associated with connective tissue diseases and chronic, progressive, or recurrent AION [25-27]. NAION also has been associated with the use of sildenafil (Viagra) for erectile dysfunction [28], after oxymetazoline nasal spray use [29], and following refractive corneal surgery (LASIK) [30].

Posterior ischemic optic neuropathy (PION) occurs rarely and usually in one of three settings: 1) hypotension associated with major surgery or hemodynamic shock [31]; 2) giant cell arteritis [32]; or 3) associated with systemic vascular disease. When PION occurs in the absence of an obvious precipitating cause, it should be considered a diagnosis of exclusion [33].

MAIN CLINICAL FEATURES

Vision loss is abrupt, painless, and often noted on awakening [34]. Visual field defects tend to have an altitudinal or arcuate pattern in NAION. Recurrences in the same eye are rare [26,35,36]. Fifty percent to 60% of patients have a stable loss of vision, approximately 10% have some progression over the initial 6 weeks, and the remaining 30-40% show some improvement over a few months [37-39].

HISTORY AND EXAMINATION

In addition to best-corrected visual acuity, careful pupil evaluation and formal visual field evaluation should be performed. Ophthalmoscopic study of the optic disc is aimed at identifying the classic acute findings of AION (disc edema, peripapillary hemorrhages, and peripapillary nerve fiber layer infarctions) or chronic findings (sectorial atrophy or hemiatrophy of the disc). If only one eye is involved, the finding of a small C/D ratio in the fellow eye is an important observation consistent with the diagnosis of NAION. Interestingly, a subset of patients with

---

Box 1-1   Differential Diagnosis of Nonarteritic Anterior Ischemic Optic Neuropathy (Optic Disc Swelling with Visual Loss)

Optic neuritis (papillitis)
Neuroretinitis
Amiodarone optic neuropathy
Partial central retinal vein occlusion
Ischemic ocular syndrome
Diabetic papillopathy
Optic nerve drusen
Optic nerve meningioma
Hypertensive disc edema
Leber's hereditary optic neuropathy
Infiltrative optic neuropathies (e.g., sarcoid, lymphoma, other metastatic cancer)

NAION has nonspecific macular edema. This finding can be very subtle at first but usually declares itself by the formation of a small partial macular star figure. It may be that this minority of patients with macular edema comprise the majority of those who improve spontaneously [40].

INVESTIGATIONS

The major investigations are aimed at documenting the risk factors for atherogenesis as discussed in the section on Overview and Etiology. Documentation of sleep apnea may be important in ultimately protecting the fellow eye, but this is only speculation at present [11]. If giant cell arteritis is suspected, a more specific evaluation is recommended (see Chapter 14).

Hyperhomocysteinemia is a risk factor for atherothrombosis and has been reported in patients with NAION or retinal artery occlusion [41].

Carotid artery evaluation is not a usual part of the NAION evaluation, although isolated reports of ipsilateral high grade carotid stenosis [42] and carotid artery hypoplasia associated with NAION have been published [43]. An exception should be made if the NAION was preceded by transient monocular blindness or if retinal emboli are seen [24].

DIFFERENTIAL DIAGNOSIS

The main differential diagnosis is between the arteritic and nonarteritic forms of AION. Other causes of optic disc edema with vision loss should be kept in mind (Box 1-1).

TREATMENT
Medical
Aspirin

In a retrospective clinical preliminary report by Kupersmith and colleagues, ingestion of aspirin (65-1,300 mg) more than once a week halved the risk of second-eye involvement in patients with NAION [44]. One report suggests that aspirin use does not affect the visual outcome after NAION has occurred [45]. Other retrospective studies suggest a positive effect, possibly short term, but prospective controlled studies are not available [46,47]. However, given the overwhelming data on aspirin use and the prevention of heart attack and stroke [48,49], I (RT) recommend its use in patients with NAION as long as no contraindications are present.

Steroids
The efficacy of corticosteroids in treating NAION is unproved. Theoretically, their use might have a salutary effect on optic disc edema in the early stages of ischemia. One author advocates steroid use if the patient is seen within the first 48 hours of vision loss [50]. A recent review of seven clinical trials encompassing 453 patients with acute ischemic stroke concludes that not enough evidence is available to assess the use of corticosteroids in this condition [51].

Calcium Channel Blockers
Suggestive evidence for the salutary effects of calcium channel blockers in the treatment of normal tension glaucoma and vasospastic amaurosis fugax raises the possibility of their use in NAION [52] (see also Chapter 5). However, clinical data are not yet available on this matter.

Topical Beta Blockers
Increased intraocular pressure plays a role in some cases of NAION [7, 8] and may cause decreased perfusion pressure of the optic disc [53]. In experiments with cats, Bennun and Nemet [54] found that optic disc blood flow was reduced when intraocular pressure increased to 30-45% of mean systemic blood pressure. Betaxolol, a selective beta-adrenergic blocker, seemed to have vasorelaxing effects on the optic disc circulation in patients with normal tension glaucoma [55]. Theoretically, therefore, the use of topical betaxolol in treating and possibly preventing NAION has merit as long as systemic hypotension is not amplified.

Levodopa
Johnson and coworkers found a small but significant improvement in the visual acuities of patients with NAION when treated with a combination of levodopa, 100 mg, and carbidopa, 25 mg, three times per day [56]. Visual fields and color vision, however, showed no improvement. I have treated four NAION patients with this drug combination up to five times per day. No subjective improvement was noted by any of them, nor could I document improvement in visual acuities, color vision, or visual fields.

Other Agents
Although not studied for treatment of NAION, acetazolamide [57] and pentoxifylline [58] have been shown to improve retinal circulation in humans. These drugs are therefore of potential, but unproved, use in treating NAION.

The use of IV norepinephrine to increase blood pressure in three patients with NAION resulted in temporary improvement in vision [59].

The alpha-2 adrenergic blocker brimonidine tartrate (Alphagan) was reported to have neuroprotective qualities in a rat model of transient ischemia-induced retinal ganglion cell death [60], and thus would seem to have potential clinical use in the acute phases of NAION. Although one study showed that brimonidine caused porcine ciliary arteries to constrict [61], another study performed in healthy humans showed no negative hemodynamic effects by scanning laser ophthalmoscopy and color doppler imaging [62]. A small retrospective study of the use of brimonidine tartrate in NAION found no clinical effect [63]. However, based on theoretical grounds and its safety and tolerability profile over the short term, I have used brimonidine tartrate in almost all patients with acute NAION since the drug has been available.

If macular edema accompanies NAION, I prescribe Voltaren (diclofenac sodium) eye drops four times a day until the disc swelling and macular edema have resolved [40].

Hyperhomocysteinemia can be treated with vitamins B_{12} and B_6 and folic acid [64].

Surgical Treatment

The initial report by Sergott and coworkers suggested that optic nerve sheath decompression (ONSD) improved vision in progressive AION [65]. This report was followed by a flurry of uncontrolled and anecdotal reports supporting and refuting the efficacy of this procedure. These responses culminated in the Ischemic Optic Neuropathy Decompression Trial, a randomized, multicenter controlled clinical trial sponsored by the National Eye Institute that compared ONSD to no treatment in patients with NAION. The study was discontinued when ONSD was found not effective and possibly harmful in patients with ischemic optic neuropathy [38]. Indeed, 24% of the surgery group had lost three or more lines of vision after a 6-month follow-up period compared to 12% in the nonsurgical group. Therefore, ONSD is contraindicated in patients with NAION.

CASE STUDY

A 44-year-old man was diagnosed with acute NAION affecting the right eye in October 1992. In March 1996, the left eye was affected. Examination disclosed acuities of 20/15 – 2 OD and 20/25 + 2 OS. He missed one Ishihara color plate with the right eye and six with the left eye. A relative afferent pupillary defect was not observed. Intraocular pressures were 24 mm Hg OD and 22 mm Hg OS. The right optic disc (Figure 1-1) showed sectorial pallor of the upper temporal quadrant. The left optic disc (Figure 1-2) showed moderate disc edema. Corresponding visual fields are shown in Figures 1-3 and 1-4.

Comment

This case study is a good example of the pseudo-Foster Kennedy syndrome, with the right eye having been affected about $3^1/2$ years before the left. Note that the patient's intraocular pressure is borderline high. Note also that there is a small-to-absent C/D ratio in the right eye. Both

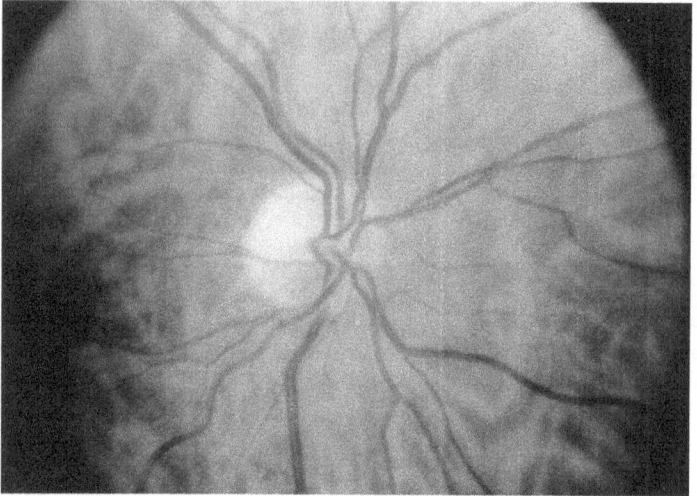

Fig. 1-1   Pseudo-Foster Kennedy's syndrome. Right optic disc showing atrophy of upper temporal quadrant.

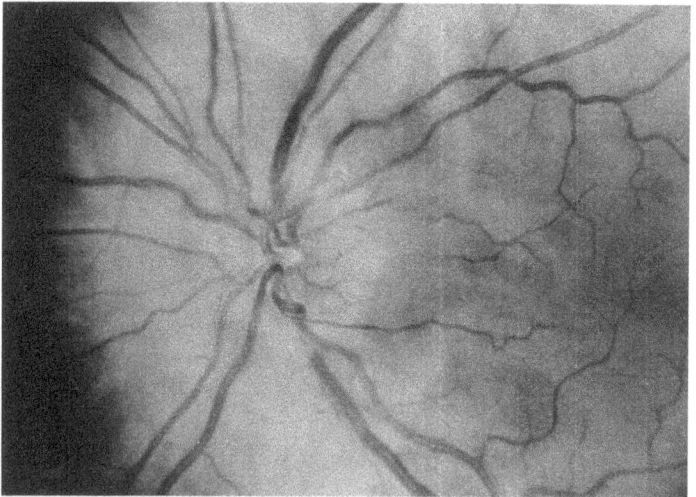

Fig. 1-2   Pseudo-Foster Kennedy's syndrome. Left optic disc showing acute disc edema characteristic of nonarteritic anterior ischemic optic neuropathy.

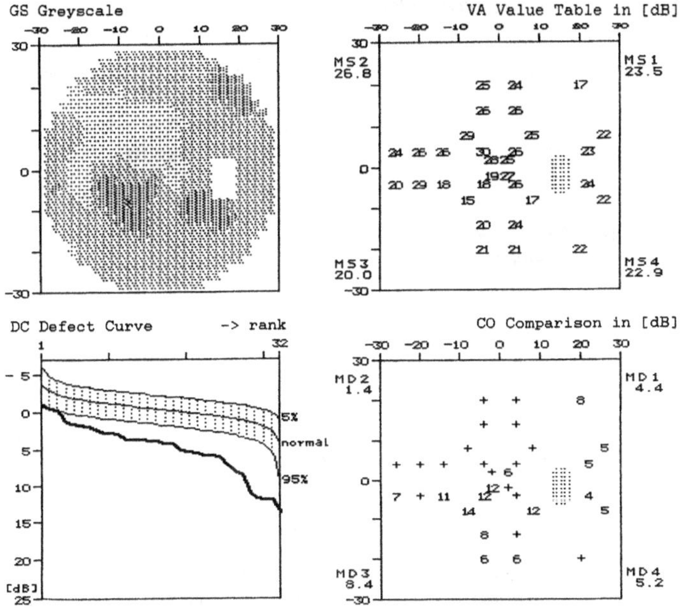

Fig. 1-3 Pseudo-Foster Kennedy's syndrome. Octopus 123 G1X (InterZeag, Switzerland) visual field of right eye showing subtle inferior altitudinal defect.

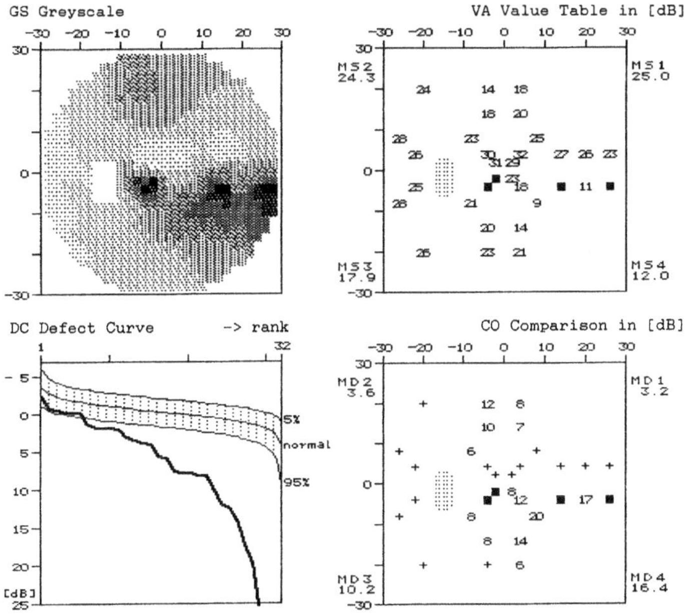

Fig. 1-4 Pseudo-Foster Kennedy's syndrome. Octopus 123 G1X (InterZeag, Switzerland) visual field of left eye showing denser inferior nasal defect.

of these are risk factors for NAION as noted in the section on Overview and Etiology.

This patient was treated with betaxolol (Betoptic S) eye drops in both eyes and one adult aspirin per day and scheduled for a follow-up examination in 1 month.

REFERENCES

1. Miller GR, Smith JL. Ischemic optic neuropathy. Am J Ophthalmol 1966;62:103.
2. Boghen D, Glaser J. Ischemic optic neuropathy: the clinical profile and natural history. Brain 1975;98:689.
3. Awai T. Studies on the pathogenesis of anterior ischemic optic neuropathy. Neuroophthalmology 1986;6:329.
4. Salomon O, Huna-Baron R, Kurtz S, et al. Analysis of prothrombotic and vascular risk factors in patients with nonarteritic anterior ischemic optic neuropathy. Ophthalmol 1999;106:739.
5. Chung SM, Gay CA, McCrary JA III. Nonarteritic ischemic optic neuropathy: the impact of tobacco use. Ophthalmology 1994;101:779.
6. Hayreh SS, Joos KM, Podhajsky PA, et al. Systemic diseases associated with nonarteritic anterior ischemic optic neuropathy. Am J Ophthalmol 1994;118:766.
7. Tomsak RL, Remler BF. Anterior ischemic optic neuropathy and increased intraocular pressure. J Clin Neuroophthalmol 1989;9:11.
8. Katz B, Weinreb RN, Wheeler T, et al. Anterior ischemic optic neuropathy and intraocular pressure. Br J Ophthalmol 1990;74:99.
9. Talks SJ, Chong NHV, Gibson JM, et al. Fibrinogen, cholesterol and smoking as risk factors for non-arteritic anterior ischemic optic neuropathy. Eye 1995;9:85.
10. Hayreh SS, Zimmerman B, Podhajsky P, Alward WLM. Nocturnal arterial hypotension and its role in optic nerve head and ocular ischemic disorders. Am J Ophthalmol 1994;117:603.
11. Mojon DS, Hedges III TR, Ehrenberg B, et al. Association between sleep apnea syndrome and nonarteritic anterior ischemic optic neuropathy. Arch Ophthalmol 2002;120:601.
12. Hayreh SS. Anterior ischemic optic neuropathy: trouble waiting to happen. Ophthalmol 2000;107:407.
13. Fiet RH, Tomsak RL, Ellenberger C. Structural factors in the pathogenesis of ischemic optic neuropathy. Am J Ophthalmol 1984;98:105.
14. Beck RW, Savino PJ, Repka MX, et al. Optic disc structure in anterior ischemic optic neuropathy. Ophthalmology 1984;91:1334.
15. Jonas JB, Xu L. Optic disc morphology in eyes after nonarteritic anterior ischemic optic neuropathy. Invest Ophthalmol Vis Sci 1993;34:2260.
16. Burde RM. Optic disc risk factors for nonarteritic anterior ischemic optic neuropathy. Am J Ophthalmol 1993;116:759.
17. Newman NJ, Scherer R, Langenberg P, et al. The fellow eye in NAION: report from the ischemic optic neuropathy decompression trial follow-up study. Am J Ophthalmol 2002;134:317.
18. Arnold AC, Hepler RS, Hamilton DR, et al. Magnetic resonance imaging of the brain in nonarteritic ischemic optic neuropathy. J Neuroophthalmol 1995;15:158.
19. Spedick MJ, Tomsak RL. Ischemic optic neuropathy following secondary intraocular lens implantation. J Clin Neuroophthalmol 1984;4:255.
20. Waybright EA, Selhorst JB, Combs J. Anterior ischemic optic neuropathy with internal carotid occlusion. Am J Ophthalmol 1982;93:42.
21. Sweeney PJ, Breuer AC, Lederman RL, et al. Ischemic optic neuropathy: a complication of coronary artery bypass surgery. Neurology 1982;32:560.

22. Tomsak RL. Ischemic optic neuropathy associated with retinal embolism. Am J Ophthalmol 1985;99:590.

23. Fry CL, Carter JE, Kanter MC, et al. Anterior ischemic optic neuropathy is not associated with carotid artery atherosclerosis. Stroke 1993;24:539.

24. Mekari-Sabbagh ON, Foroozan R, Danesh-Meyer H, Savino PJ. Non-arteritic anterior ischemic optic neuropathy with retinal emboli. Neuroophthalmology 2001;25:123.

25. Slavin ML. Chronic asymptomatic ischemic optic neuropathy: a report of two cases in adults with diabetes mellitus. J Clin Neuroophthalmol 1987;7:198.

26. Borchert M, Lessell S. Progressive and recurrent nonarteritic anterior ischemic optic neuropathy. Am J Ophthalmol 1988;106:443.

27. Hamed LM, Purvin V, Rosenberg M. Recurrent anterior ischemic optic neuropathy in young adults. J Clin Neuroophthalmol 1988;8:239.

28. Pomeranz HD, Smith KH, Hart WM Jr, Egan RA. Sildenafil-associated nonarteritic anterior ischemic optic neuropathy. Ophthalmol 2002;109:584.

29. Fivgas GD, Newman NJ. Anterior ischemic optic neuropathy following the use of a nasal decongestant. Am J Ophthalmol 1999;127:104.

30. Lee AG, Kohnen T, Ebner R, et al. Optic neuropathy associated with laser in situ keratomileusis. J Cataract Refract Surg 2000;26:1581.

31. Alexandrakis G, Lam BL. Bilateral posterior ischemic optic neuropathy after spinal surgery. Am J Ophthalmol 1999;127:354.

32. Sadda SR, Nee M, Miller NR, et al. Clinical spectrum of posterior ischemic optic neuropathy. Am J Ophthalmol 2001;132:743.

33. Sadun AA, Dao J. Annual review in neuro-ophthalmology. The anterior visual pathways. Part two. J Neuroophthalmol 1994;14:234.

34. Hayreh SS, Zimmerman MB, Podhajsky P, et al. Nocturnal arterial hypotension and its role in optic nerve head and ocular ischemic disorders. Am J Ophthalmol 1994;117:603.

35. Lavin PJM, Ellenberger C. Recurrent ischemic optic neuropathy. Neuroophthalmology 1982;3:193.

36. Hayreh SS, Podhajsky PA, Zimmerman B. Ipsilateral recurrence of nonarteritic anterior ischemic optic neuropathy. Am J Ophthalmol 2001;132:734.

37. Yee D, Selky AK, Purvin VA. Outcomes of surgical and nonsurgical management of nonarteritic anterior ischemic optic neuropathy. Trans Am Ophthalmol Soc 1993;91:227.

38. Ischemic Optic Neuropathy Decompression Trial Research Group. Optic nerve decompression surgery for nonarteritic anterior ischemic optic neuropathy (NAION) is not effective and may be harmful. JAMA 1995;273:625.

39. Arnold AC, Hepler RS. Natural history of nonarteritic anterior ischemic optic neuropathy. J Neuroophthalmol 1994;14:66.

40. Tomsak RL, Zakov ZN. Nonarteritic anterior ischemic optic neuropathy with macular edema: visual improvement and fluorescein angiographic characteristics. J Neuroophthalmol 1998;18:166.

41. Pianka P, Almog Y, Man O, et al. Hyperhomocystinemia in patients with nonarteritic anterior ischemic optic neuropathy, central retinal artery occlusion, and central retinal vein occlusion. Ophthalmol 2000;107:1588.

42. Mendez MV, Wijman CA, Matjucha IC, Menzoian JO. Carotid endarterectomy in a patient with anterior ischemic neuropathy. J Vasc Surg 1998;28:1107.

43. Horowitz J, Melamud A, Sela L, Hod Y, Geyer O. Internal carotid artery hypoplasia presenting as anterior ischemic optic neuropathy. Am J Ophthalmol 2001;131:673.

44. Kupersmith MJ, Frohman LP, Sanderson MC, et al. Aspirin reduces second eye anterior ischemic optic neuropathy. Ophthalmology 1995;102(Suppl):104.

45. Botelho PJ, Johnson LN, Arnold AC. The effect of aspirin on the visual outcome of nonarteritic anterior ischemic optic neuropathy. Am J Ophthalmol 1996;121:450.

46. Beck RW, Hayreh SS, Podhajsky PA, et al. Aspirin therapy in nonarteritic anterior ischemic optic neuropathy. Am J Ophthalmol 1997;123:212.

47. Salomon O, Huna-Baron R, Steinberg DM, et al. Role of aspirin in reducing the frequency of second eye involvement in patients with non-arteritic anterior ischemic optic neuropathy. Eye 2000;13(part 3a):357.

48. Dalen JE. Selective COX-2 inhibitors, NSAIDs, aspirin and myocardial infarction (editorial). Arch Int Med 2002;162:1091.

49. Hankey GJ, Sudlow CLM, Dunbabin DW. Thienopyridine derivatives (ticlopidine, clopidogrel) versus aspirin for preventing stroke and other serious vascular events in high risk vascular patients. Coch Lib 2002;1.

50. Kay MC. Ischemic optic neuropathy. Neurol Clin 1991;9:115.

51. Qizilbash N, Lewington SL, Lopez-Arrieta JM. Corticosteroids for acute ischemic stroke. Cochrane Database Syst Rev 2000;2:CD000064.

52. Winterkorn JMS, Kupersmith MJ, Wirtschafter JD, et al. Brief report: treatment of vasospastic amaurosis fugax with calcium-channel blockers. N Engl J Med 1993;329:396.

53. Hayreh SS. Progress in the understanding of the vascular etiology of glaucoma. Curr Opin Ophthalmol 1994:5:26.

54. Bennun J, Nemet P. Intraocular pressure and blood flow of the optic disk: a fluorescent blood cell angiography study. Surv Ophthalmol 1995;39(Suppl 1):S33.

55. Harris A, Spaeth GL, Sergott RC, et al. Retrobulbar arterial hemodynamic effects of betaxolol and timolol in normal-tension glaucoma. Am J Ophthalmol 1995;120:168.

56. Johnson LN, Gould TJ, Krohel GB. Effect of levodopa and carbidopa on recovery of visual function in patients with nonarteritic anterior ischemic optic neuropathy of longer than six month's duration. Am J Ophthalmol 1996;121:77.

57. Rassam SMB, Patel V, Kohner EM. The effect of acetazolamide on the retinal circulation. Eye 1993;7:697.

58. Sonkin PL, Kelly LW, Sinclair SH, et al. Pentoxifylline increases retinal capillary blood flow velocity in patients with diabetes. Arch Ophthalmol 1993;111:1647.

59. Kollarits CR, McCarthy RW, Corrie WS, et al. Norepinephrine therapy of ischemic optic neuropathy. J Clin Neuroophthalmol 1981;1:283.

60. Lafuente MP, Villegas-Perez MP, Mayor S, et al. Neuroprotective effects of brimonidine against transient ischemia-induced retinal ganglion cell death: a dose response in vivo study. Exp Eye Res 2002;74:181.

61. Wikberg-Matsson A, Simonsen U. Potent alpha (2A) adrenoreceptor mediated vasoconstriction by brimonidine in porcine ciliary arteries. Invest Ophthalmol Vis Sci 2001;42:2049.

62. Jonescu-Cuypers CP, Harris A, Ishii Y, et al. Effect of brimonidine tartrate on ocular hemodynamics in healthy volunteers. J Ocul Pharmacol Ther 2001;17:199.

63. Fazzone HE, Kupersmith MJ. Does topical brimonidine tartrate help NAION? Platform presentation, North American Neuro-ophthalmological Society Meeting, Copper Mountain Colorado, 2002.

64. Willems FF, Aengevaeren WR, Boers GH, et al. Coronary endothelial function in hyperhomocystinemia: improvement after treatment with folic acid and cobalamin in patients with coronary artery disease. J Am Coll Cardiol 2002;40:766.

65. Sergott RC, Cohen MS, Bosley TM, et al. Optic nerve decompression may improve the progressive form of nonarteritic ischemic optic neuropathy. Arch Ophthalmol 1989;107:1743.

2

Botulinum Toxin

OVERVIEW

Since the pioneering work of Scott, botulinum toxin type A (BOTOX, [Allergan, Inc., Irvine, CA]) (BTX) has been used therapeutically for more than 15 years [1]. Seven toxins (A, B, C, D, E, F, G) are produced by the bacterium *Clostridium botulinum*. Toxin A has the highest specific activity for humans, but types B, E, and F are also neurotoxic in humans; types C and D are pathogenic in birds and mammals. Toxin F has a shorter duration of effect — approximately 1 month — in humans. BTX works by inhibiting release of acetylcholine from cholinergic nerve endings at the neuromuscular junction. Its intracellular target is SNAP-25, a synaptosome-associated protein required for the release of vesicles containing acetylcholine. BTX permanently disables the SNAP-25 molecule by cleaving it. This binding is accompanied by loss of junctional acetylcholine receptors. The binding is irreversible and takes approximately 24 hours to complete [2-4].

NEURO-OPHTHALMIC USES OF BOTULINUM TOXIN

See Box 2-1 for a list of the neuro-ophthalmic uses of BTX.

DOSAGES AND ADMINISTRATION

BTX is provided frozen and lyophilized in 100-U vials. The medication is reconstituted just before use with sterile, 0.9% NaCl (normal saline) for injection. A recent study suggests that using normal saline with preservative results in less painful injections and may add to its stability [5]. A preinjection Schirmer's test for baseline tear production is recommended, as are artificial tears and lubricating ointments at night for any patient receiving BTX to eyelids or eye muscles [6].

Botulinum toxin type B is now being marketed (MYOBLOC; Elan Pharmaceuticals, Dublin, Ireland) for treatment of cervical dystonia. Botulinum toxin type B is antigenically different from type A and works by a different mechanism and thus is a possible alternative treatment for essential blepharospasm, if resistance to BOTOX develops [7].

Strabismus and Diplopia

The usual method for treating strabismus and diplopia is to inject 2.5-5.0 U of toxin directly into the selected muscle under electromyographic (EMG) control following the protocol of Scott [1]. The maximal effect

---

Box 2-1   Uses of Botulinum Toxin in Neuro-Ophthalmology

Eye movement disturbances
Strabismus
Paralytic strabismus
Diplopia following retinal detachment surgery
Nystagmus or oscillopsia
Thyroid-related ophthalmopathy
Benign essential blepharospasm
Hemifacial spasm
Eye-opening apraxia
Aberrant regeneration of the seventh cranial nerve
Lower lid entropion
Corneal ulcer and exposure
Other dystonias
Headache
Thyroid-related eyelid retraction

Sources: Jankovic J, Schwartz K. Response and immunoresistance to botulinum toxin injections. Neurology 1995;45:1743; Osako M, Keltner JL. Botulinum A toxin (Oculinum) in ophthalmology. Surv Ophthalmol 1991;36:28; Mauriello JA, Wagner RS, Mostafavi R, et al. Oculinum therapy: its use in neuro-ophthalmology. In Tusa RJ, Newman SA (eds). Neuro-Ophthalmological Disorders. Diagnostic Work-up and Therapy. New York: Dekker, 1995;451; Hassan SM, Jennekens FGI, Veldman H. Botulinum toxin-induced myopathy in the rat. Brain 1995;118:533; Uddin JM, Davies PD. Treatment of upper eyelid retraction associated with thyroid eye disease with subconjunctival botulinum toxin injections. Ophthalmology 2002;109:1183; and Silberstein SD, Mathew N, Saper J, Jenkin S. Botulinum toxin type A as a migraine preventive treatment: for the Botox Migraine Clinical Research Group. Headache 2000;40:445.

occurs in 2-5 days and lasts 2-3 months. See Rosenbaum [8], Mauriello and coworkers [9], Huber [10], Scott [11], and Dunn and coworkers [12] for further details.

Nystagmus

In our experience, the side effects have outweighed the benefits. See Chapter 7 for further discussion.

The treatment of nystagmus and oscillopsia with BTX has received mixed reviews. Individual antagonistic pairs of muscles can be injected, or the medication can be given by retrobulbar injection (≤25 U).

Benign Essential Blepharospasm and Hemifacial Spasm

BTX is usually prepared at a concentration of 25 U/mL (i.e., 2.5 U/0.1 ml). To treat benign essential blepharospasm (BEB) and hemifacial spasm, 2.5-5.0 U is injected at selected sites in the eyelids and face (Figures 2-1 and 2-2). The patients are re-evaluated 2 weeks after injection and further injections are done if needed. In one series, the duration of effect was 12-14 weeks for BEB and 16-18 weeks for hemifacial spasm. These authors noted that BTX injections had no effect in 3-7% of patients and that 3% had an initial good response but no response to further injections [9]. This latter finding may be due to the production of neutralizing antibodies against BTX [2, 13]. The concomitant use of oral cyproheptadine (Periactin) may facilitate the effects of BTX [9]. See Angibaud et al. [14], Lorentz [15], and Ainsworth and Kraft [16] for further discussion.

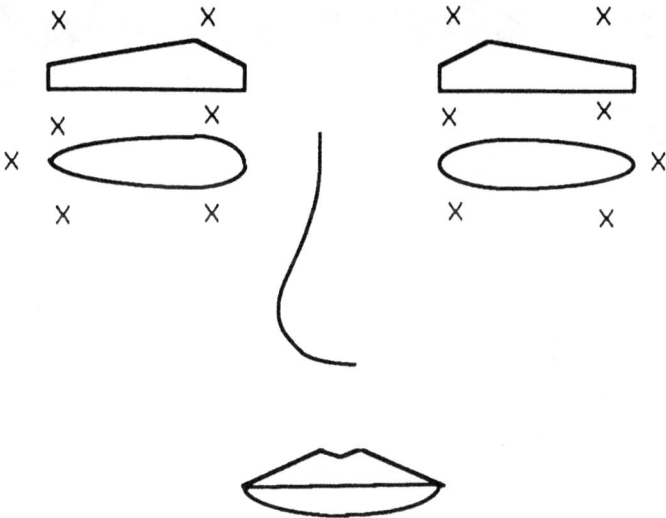

Fig. 2-1 Possible sites of botulinum toxin type A injection for benign essential blepharospasm. (Reproduced with permission from Osako M, Keltner JL. Botulinum A toxin [Oculinum] in ophthalmology. Surv Ophthalmol 1991;36:28.)

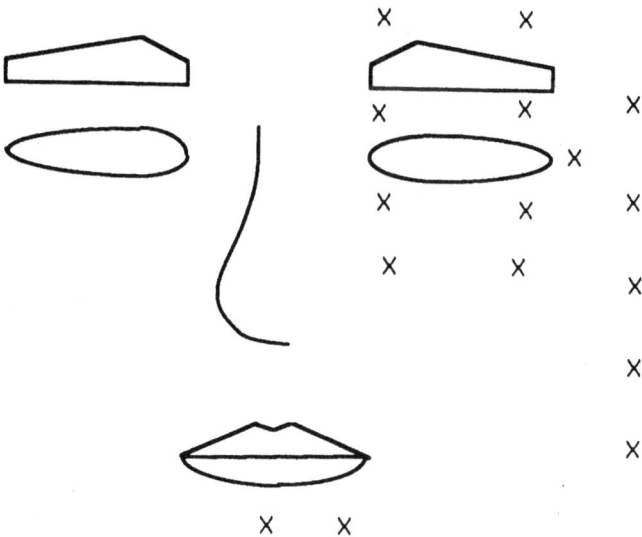

Fig. 2-2 Possible sites of botulinum toxin type A injection for left hemifacial spasm. (Reproduced with permission from Osako M, Keltner JL. Botulinum A toxin [Oculinum] in ophthalmology. Surv Ophthalmol 1991;36:28.)

> **Box 2-2   Adverse Effects of Neuro-Ophthalmologic Uses of Botulinum Toxin**
>
> Ptosis
> Diplopia
> Dry-eye symptoms
> Filamentary keratitis
> Excessive tearing
> Excessive weakening of injected muscle
> Brow ptosis
> Entropion or ectropion
> Lower facial weakness
> Eyelid necrosis
> Lid or facial hemorrhage
> Ocular perforation
> Retrobulbar hemorrhage
> Myotoxicity (rat model)
> Antigenic sensitization leading to decreased effect of subsequent injections

Sources: Jankovic J, Schwartz K. Response and immunoresistance to botulinum toxin injections. Neurology 1995;45:1743; Osako M, Keltner JL. Botulinum A toxin (Oculinum) in ophthalmology. Surv Ophthalmol 1991;36:28; Tomsak RL, Remler BF, Averbuch-Heller L, et al. Unsatisfactory treatment of acquired nystagmus with retrobulbar injection of botulinum toxin. Am J Ophthalmol 1995;119:489; Borodic G, Johnson E, Goodnough M, et al. Botulinum toxin therapy, immunologic resistance, and problems with available materials. Neurology 1996;46:26; Lorentz IT. Treatment of hemifacial spasm with botulinum toxin. J Clin Neurosci 1995;2:132; Botulinum toxin for ocular muscle disorders. Med Lett 1990;32:100; Hassan SM, Jennekens FGI, Veldman H. Botulinum toxin-induced myopathy in the rat. Brain 1995;118:533; and Savino PJ, Maus M. Botulinum toxin therapy. Neurol Clin 1991;9:205.

COMPLICATIONS

Although BTX, on a molecule-by-molecule basis, is more than 2 million times as toxic as cobra venom and about 10^{11} times as toxic as cyanide, clinical botulism has not been reported after human therapeutic use [17]. This is because the estimated toxic dose is 40 U/kg in humans [9]. However, a remote, subclinical effect of BTX can be demonstrated by EMG in muscles distant from the administration site [18]. For a list of possible complications associated with BTX, see Box 2-2.

REFERENCES

1. Scott AB. Botulinum toxin injection of eye muscles to correct strabismus. Trans Am Ophthalmol Soc 1981;79:734.
2. Jankovic J, Schwartz K. Response and immunoresistance to botulinum toxin injections. Neurology 1995;45:1743.
3. Bell MS, Vermeulen LC, Sperling KB. Pharmacotherapy with botulinum toxin: Harnessing natures most potent neurotoxin. Pharmacotherapy 2000;20:1079.
4. Osako M, Keltner JL. Botulinum A toxin (Oculinum) in ophthalmology. Surv Ophthalmol 1991;36:28.
5. Alam M, Dover JS, Arndt KA. Pain associated with injection of botulinum A exotoxin reconstituted using isotonic sodium chloride with and without preservative: a double-blind, randomized controlled trial. Arch Dermatol 2002;138:510. New York: Dekker, 1995;451.
6. Tomsak RL, Remler BF, Averbuch-Heller L, et al. Unsatisfactory treatment of acquired nystagmus with retrobulbar injection of botulinum toxin. Am J Ophthalmol 1995;119:489.

7. Lew ME, Brashear A, Factor, S. The safety and efficacy of botulinum toxin type B in the treatment of patients with cervical dystonia: Summary of three controlled clinical trials. Neurology 2000;55(Suppl 5):S29.

8. Rosenbaum AL. The current use of botulinum toxin therapy in strabismus. Arch Ophthalmol 1996;114:213.

9. Mauriello JA, Wagner RS, Mostafavi R, et al. Oculinum therapy: its use in neuro-ophthalmology. In Tusa RJ, Newman SA (eds), Neuro-Ophthalmological Disorders. Diagnostic Work-up and Therapy. New York: Dekker, 1995;45.

10. Huber A. Botulinum toxin in the treatment of paralytic strabismus. Neuroophthalmology 1995;16:11.

11. Scott AB. Botulinum treatment of strabismus following retinal detachment surgery. Arch Ophthalmol 1990;108:509.

12. Dunn WJ, Arnold AC, O'Connor PS. Botulinum toxin for the treatment of dysthyroid ocular myopathy. Ophthalmology 1986;93:470.

13. Sankhla C, Jankovic J, Duane D. Variability of the immunologic and clinical response in dystonic patients immunoresistant to botulinum toxin injections. Mov Disord 1998;13:150.

14. Angibaud G, Moreau MS, Rascol O, et al. Treatment of hemifacial spasm with botulinum toxin: value of preinjection electromyography abnormalities for predicting postinjection lower facial paresis. Eur Neurol 1995;35:43.

15. Lorentz IT. Treatment of hemifacial spasm with botulinum toxin. J Clin Neurosci 1995;2:132.

16. Ainsworth JR, Kraft SP. Long-term changes in duration of relief with botulinum toxin treatment of essential blepharospasm and hemifacial spasm. Ophthalmology 1995;102:2036.

17. Davis LE. Botulinum toxin: from poison to medicine. West J Med 1993;158:25.

18. Sanders DB, Massey EW, Buckley EG. Botulinum toxin for blepharospasm: single-fiber EMG studies. Neurology 1986;36:545.
    Savino PJ, Maus M. Botulinum toxin therapy. Neurol Clin 1991;9:205.

3

Diplopia

OVERVIEW AND ETIOLOGY

Diplopia, or double vision, usually results from disorders of the extraocular muscles, the cranial nerves that supply these muscles, or the central neural pathways that coordinate eye movements (Box 3-1). Monocular diplopia is almost always caused by a refractive or optical error in the eye.

HISTORY

Patient history is extremely important in ascertaining the cause of the diplopia. Answers to the following questions will lead the examiner in the right direction long before the examination is performed.

1. *Is the diplopia monocular or binocular?* Monocular diplopia is usually reported as a ghost image or halos and never as discrete images. Monocular diplopia rarely presents as a psychogenic visual symptom.

Remember that monocular diplopia can affect both eyes but is, with few exceptions, due to a refractive or optical error [1,2]. Retinal causes for monocular diplopia are debatable [3,4]. A pinhole device always improves the monocular diplopia — or resolves it completely — if the diplopia has an optical cause.

Binocular diplopia is almost always a result of misalignment of the visual axes caused by ocular motor imbalance. Binocular diplopia can

---

Box 3-1   Major Forms of Diplopia

Disorders of the eye muscles
Ocular myasthenia, thyroid eye disease, muscle entrapment from orbital trauma, orbital myositis

Disorders of cranial nerves supplying eye muscles (CN III, IV, and VI)
Trauma, microvascular ischemia, compression

Disorders of central pathways coordinating eye movement
Internuclear ophthalmoplegia, divergence insufficiency, skew deviation, convergence insufficiency, decompensated strabismus

Disorders of the optical system of the eye (monocular diplopia)
Nuclear lens sclerosis, uncorrected refractive error, corneal disease, pseudophakia with decentered lens, peripheral iridectomy

Disorders with unclear or combined etiologies
Chronic progressive external ophthalmoplegia (rarely have diplopia)

Box 3-2   Common Causes of Horizontal Diplopia

Acquired esotropia deviations
Sixth cranial nerve palsies
Tight medial rectus from thyroid-related ophthalmopathy
Blowout fracture of medial orbit with medial rectus entrapment
Ocular myasthenia
Spasm of convergence
Divergence insufficiency

Acquired exotropia deviations
Third cranial nerve palsies
Internuclear ophthalmoplegia with exotropia
Convergence insufficiency
Decompensated strabismus

Box 3-3   Common Causes of Vertical Diplopia

Third cranial nerve palsy
Fourth cranial nerve palsy
Thyroid-related ophthalmopathy with tight inferior rectus
Ocular myasthenia
Skew deviation
Blowout fracture of orbital floor with inferior rectus entrapment

---

also result from spectacle correction for large differences in refractive error between eyes (anisometropia), which leads to induced prism when not looking through the optical centers of the lenses (induced anisophoria) [5].

2. *Is the diplopia horizontal or vertical?* Horizontal deviations indicate either esotropia or exotropia (Box 3-2). Vertical deviations reflect dysfunction of the vertical recti or oblique muscles, the presence of skew deviation, or other supranuclear vertical gaze disturbance (Box 3-3).

3. *Is the diplopia worse at near or far distances?* Diplopia from a sixth cranial nerve palsy is worse at far distances, whereas diplopia from a fourth cranial nerve palsy is usually worse at near distances. (Answers to the first three questions usually narrow the number of possibly involved muscles from eight to two.)

4. *Is the diplopia worse in right gaze or left gaze?* For example, diplopia from a right sixth cranial nerve palsy is worse when looking to the right; diplopia from a right fourth cranial nerve palsy is worse when looking to the left (Table 3-1).

5. *Is the diplopia affected by head position?* Face turns compensate for horizontal deviations. For example, a patient with a right sixth cranial nerve palsy will usually adopt a face turn to the right to place gaze out of the field of action of the paretic muscle and thus avoid diplopia. Alternatively, the patient may preferentially fixate with the paretic eye if vision in the fellow eye is subnormal [6]. Patients with fourth cranial nerve palsies tilt the head toward the opposite side to minimize diplopia. A chin-down position with a slight face turn away from the side of paresis may also be seen in these cases [7].

Table 3-1	Results of the Parks-Bielschowsky Head-Tilt Test		
Hypertropia	Worse on Gaze to:	Worse on Head Tilt to:	Paretic Muscle
Right	Right	Right	Left inferior oblique
Right	Right	Left	Right inferior rectus
Right	Left	Right	Right superior oblique
Right	Left	Left	Left superior rectus
Left	Left	Left	Right inferior oblique
Left	Left	Right	Left inferior rectus
Left	Right	Left	Left superior oblique
Left	Right	Right	Right superior rectus

Chin-up or chin-down positions are often seen in restrictive or paretic strabismus when vertically acting muscles are affected. For example, a patient with thyroid eye disease and a tight left inferior rectus might adopt a chin-up position to place the unaffected yoke muscles in downgaze. It is always helpful to review old photographs or the family photo album, which may prove that the ocular torticollis has been present for years. Therefore, in the evaluation for diplopia, "family album tomography" (a "FAT scan") should be performed before computed tomography or magnetic resonance imaging (MRI).

6. *Was the onset of the diplopia sudden or slow?* Sudden onset is seen in microvascular ischemia, trauma, and sudden expansion of an aneurysm or a cystic tumor. Slow onset of diplopia is seen in compressive lesions, myasthenia, thyroid-related ophthalmopathy, and decompensated phorias.

7. *Is the diplopia variable?* Ocular myasthenia is notoriously variable. Spasm of near reflex, convergence insufficiency, superior oblique myokymia, and other periodic and aperiodic deviations should also be considered.

8. *Does the patient have accompanying ptosis or proptosis?* Diplopia with ptosis suggests ocular myasthenia, third cranial nerve palsy, or a cavernous sinus syndrome with oculosympathetic dysfunction (Horner's syndrome, Raeder's paratrigeminal syndrome). Diplopia associated with proptosis suggests an orbital tumor or pseudotumor, thyroid-associated orbitopathy, cavernous sinus fistula, or defects in the sphenoid bone as seen in neurofibromatosis type 1.

9. *Is the patient experiencing any pain?* Painful diplopia may be seen in microvascular ischemia, aneurysm, orbital or cavernous sinus inflammation, metastases to bone, or ophthalmoplegic migraine. Thyroid-associated orbitopathy and ocular myasthenia are two common causes of painless diplopia.

EXAMINATION

Knowledge of the actions of the eye muscles (Figure 3-1) and the functional classes of eye movements (Box 3-4) is necessary to perform a diplopia evaluation. After the history is taken, the patient's glasses should be examined to see if they contain prism, which would indicate that the tendency for diplopia is longstanding and had been addressed in the past.

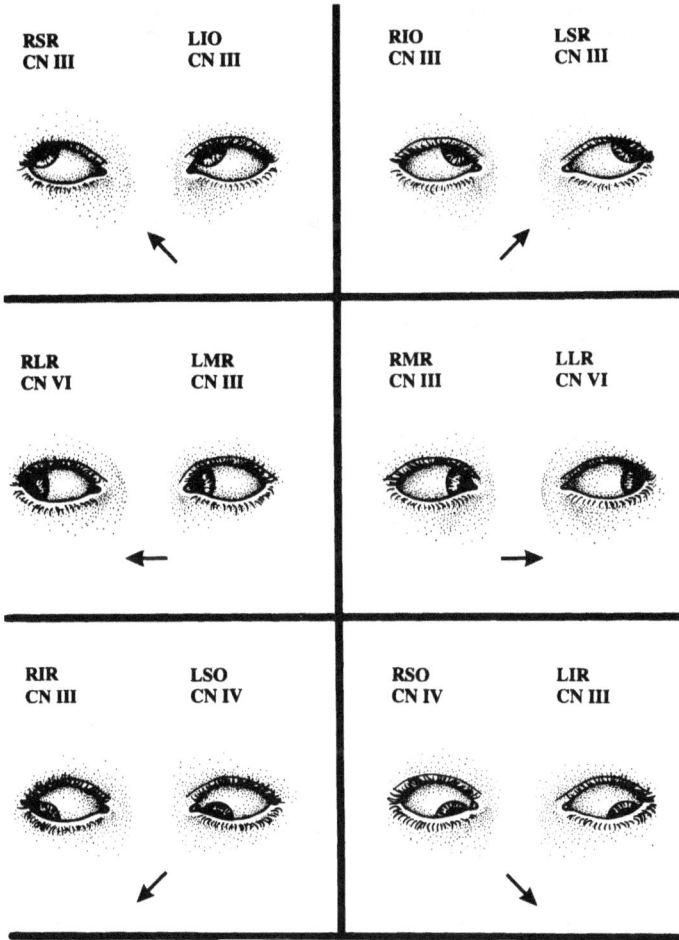

Fig. 3-1 Diagrams show primary muscle acting in various fields of gaze and cranial nerve innervation of these muscles. (RSR = right superior rectus; LIO = left inferior oblique; RIO = right inferior oblique; LSR = left superior rectus; RLR = right lateral rectus; LMR = left medical rectus; RMR = right medial rectus; LLR = left lateral rectus; RIR= right inferior rectus; LSO = left superior oblique; RSO = right superior oblique; LIR = left inferior rectus.) (Modified with permission from GK von Noorden -Maumenee's Atlas of Strabismus, 3rd ed. St. Louis: Mosby, 1977.)

Head postures are important to note: face turns are used to compensate for horizontal deviations; elevation or depression of the chin compensates for vertical deviations; and head tilts adjust for torsional deviations [6,7]. In addition to a complete eye examination, special attention should be paid to quantifying phorias and tropias. Evaluation

---

Box 3-4   Functional Classification of Human Eye Movements

Smooth pursuit: holds image of a moving target on the fovea.
Saccades: bring objects of visual interest on the fovea.
Vestibular-ocular reflex: holds visual images steady on the fovea during brief
   head rotations.
Optokinetic movements: hold visual images steady on the fovea during
   sustained head rotations.
Vergence: moves eyes in opposite directions to keep object of regard foveated
   with both eyes.
Nystagmus quick phases: direct foveas to visual objects of interest during self-
   rotation.

Source: Leigh RJ, Zee DS. The Neurology of Eye Movements, 3rd ed. Philadelphia: FA Davis, 1999.

Box 3-5   Other Tests Used in Evaluating Eye Movements

Observe steadiness of fixation with or without Frenzel lenses
Assess saccadic speed and accuracy with rapid refixations
Observe quality of pursuit
Test convergence by having subject fixate on his or her own thumb
Evaluate presence of nystagmus
Evaluate gaze-holding ability
View fundus with direct ophthalmoscope to appreciate subtle nystagmus
Measure acuity before and during horizontal and vertical head shaking (at least
   1 cycle/sec)
Assess optokinetic nystagmus
Perform caloric testing
Perform eye movement recordings

Source: Leigh RJ, Zee DS. The Neurology of Eye Movements, 3rd ed. Philadelphia: FA Davis, 1999.

---

for phorias and tropias may require the use of prisms and the alternate cover test, the use of the Maddox rod and Maddox wing, or both. This information is extremely valuable for follow-up examinations.

Corneal and facial sensation should be checked and other cranial nerves evaluated. For example, a patient with a sixth cranial nerve palsy and decreased corneal sensation on that side has a cavernous sinus syndrome or superior orbital fissure syndrome until proven otherwise. At times, diplopia needs to be evaluated with seldom-used tests such as the Lancaster red-green test. Box 3-5 lists some other tests used for evaluating eye movement disturbances and von Noorden and Campos [8] is suggested for further reference.

INVESTIGATIONS

Investigations for diplopia are tailored to the history and examination. For example, chronic progressive diplopia associated with proptosis might require thyroid function studies and orbital imaging. The evaluation of variable diplopia with ptosis would require a Tensilon test or an ice test, screening for the presence of acetylcholine-receptor antibodies, a neurologic examination, and, possibly, electromyography. An older patient with the sudden onset of painful diplopia could be symptomatic for giant cell arteritis, so acute phase reactants and a

Box 3-6   **Treatments for Binocular Diplopia**
Occlusion
Total: patch, clip-on occluder, tape
Partial: tape
Prisms
Temporary: Fresnel
Permanent: ground-in
Botulinum toxin (BTX)
Eye muscle surgery
Exercises (orthoptics)
for convergence insufficiency

temporal artery biopsy might be indicated in this case. An adult with the sudden onset of an isolated third, fourth, or sixth cranial nerve palsy may well need a glucose tolerance test or a glycosylated hemoglobin determination. In an adult or child with a chronic sixth cranial nerve palsy, an MRI is often indicated.

TREATMENT

The treatment for binocular diplopia is outlined in Box 3-6. If the patient does not wear glasses for distance, an inexpensive pair of lightly tinted sunglasses can be used to mount the Fresnel prism or occlusion tape. Total occlusion of one eye is effective, but it is the least sophisticated method and completely excludes the possibility of binocularity. When occlusion is used and one eye is paretic, it is best to cover the paretic eye; if both eyes do not move normally, occlude the eye with the greatest ophthalmoplegia for the same reason. This method allows more comfort, especially during ambulation, because the vestibulo-ocular reflex functions better in this setting. If in doubt, allow the patient a trial occlusion of one eye, then the other, in the office and let him or her choose the eye to be covered after walking around a bit.

Partial occlusion can be very useful in selected cases (Figure 3-2). For example, some patients with isolated fourth cranial nerve palsies can fuse at distance but are diplopic in a reading position. In these cases, tape occlusion of the lower half of the lens in front of the paretic eye often works well. Others with diplopia limited to down-gaze will benefit from single-vision glasses, high bifocal segments, or a symmetric base-down prism in both lenses [9].

Fresnel press-on plastic prism optics can be very helpful for patients with binocular diplopia up to 40 Δ in magnitude. These are usually available in various Δ increments from 1 to 40 Δ. I (RT) usually place the Fresnel prism in front of the paretic eye and always try to put it on only one lens of a patient's glasses to minimize blurring of vision. In certain cases cutting the prism to fit the lower or upper half of the lens can be done. In patients with a combined horizontal and vertical deviation, a nomogram is available (Figure 3-3) that allows oblique orientation of the prism axis to give both horizontal and vertical power.

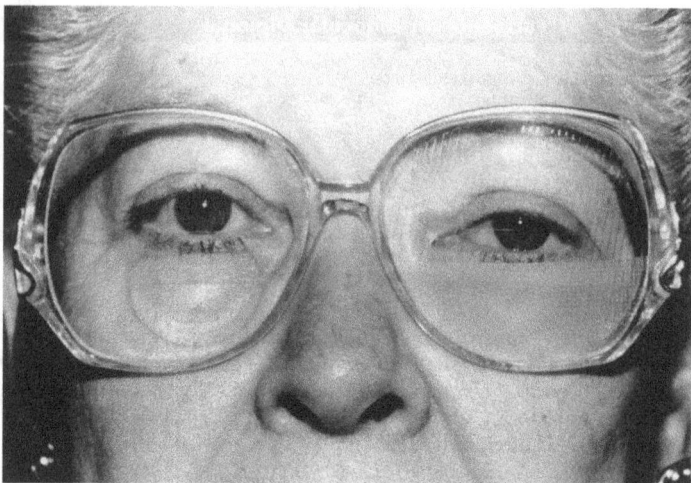

Fig. 3-2 Patient with oblique diplopia following retinal detachment surgery in the left eye. Measurements of occular misalignment were different at distance versus near. Photograph shows Fresnel prism oriented obliquely to compensate for horizontal and vertical components of deviation at distance. Bifocal portion of left lens occluded with tape to prevent diplopia when reading.

Fresnel prisms are especially useful in patients with ischemic ocular motor cranial nerve palsies and in those with diplopia from thyroid-associated orbitopathy. The latter group of patients may have diplopia that varies, usually over a period of weeks or months, and patients in the former group usually heal within a period of 90 days.

Ground-in prisms are useful for stable diplopia problems with deviations of about 12 D or less in primary position. Custom lenses are also available with multiple prisms or prism in only one part of the lens*. Box 3-7 gives some useful tips for prescribing ground-in prisms. Botulinum toxin (BTX) injections into selected eye muscles have been used to temporarily treat diplopia resulting from cranial nerve palsies, especially paralysis of the sixth nerve, thyroid eye disease, and retinal detachment surgery (see Chapter 2). The main drawbacks to treatment are the variability of effect, ptosis, and anterior segment exposure symptoms. As a rule, the salutary effect of BTX injection wears off in 3-4 months.

Discussion of the types of eye muscle surgery for the treatment of diplopia is beyond the scope of this chapter; see Helveston [10] for further information.

Eye muscle exercises (orthoptics) for the treatment of idiopathic convergence insufficiency, or that associated with head trauma, have been very successful in my experience and in the experience of others [11].

---

* Epic Labs, Inc. Waite Park, MN.

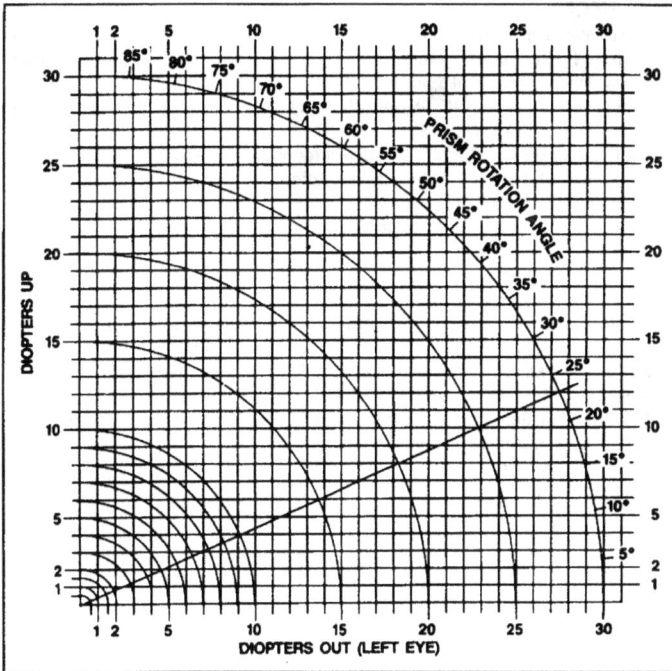

Fig. 3-3 Rotation nomogram for achieving proper vertical and horizontal prism. A. Amount of horizontal and vertical prism is determined by patient examination, and the intersection of these two values is marked on the nomogram. B. The arc nearest this point is the proper total prism power required. C. The intersection of this arc and the exact amount of vertical prism is marked and a line is drawn from the origin, through this intersection, and carried out to the prism rotation angle scale. The angle on the scale is correct orientation of the prism axis to obtain the exact vertical prism required. Note: Example is shown for measurements of 6 Δ vertical and 13 Δ horizontal. Orienting a 15-Δ prism at an angle of 23 degrees achieves 6 Δ of vertical correction and 13.8 Δ of horizontal correction. (Reproduced with permission from 3M Health Care. 3M Press-On Optics. St. Paul, MN.)

Box 3-7   Prism Prescribing Tips

Bring out maximum phoria by occluding one eye for 45 minutes.
Try intended prism in trial lenses before writing final prescription.
Use minimum amount of prism that relieves symptoms (usually $1/2$-$3/4$ of measured amount for vertical deviation).
If prism power is low and vertical is needed, place in only one lens base-up.
With large minus or plus lenses (>4 D) consider decentration to add prismatic effect.
Always recheck prism prescription with a return office visit.

Source: Adapted from Milder B, Rubin ML. The Fine Art of Prescribing Glasses Without Making a Spectacle of Yourself. Gainesville, FL: Triad, 1991;215.

REFERENCES

1. Hirst LW, Miller NR, Johnson RT. Monocular polyopia. Arch Neurol 1983;40:756.
2. Coffeen P, Guyton DL. Monocular diplopia accompanying ordinary refractive errors. Am J Ophthalmol 1988;105:451.
3. Lepore FE, Yarian DL. Monocular diplopia of retinal origin. J Clin Neuroophthalmol 1986;6:181.
4. Smith JL. Monocular diplopia. J Clin Neuroophthalmol 1986;6:184.
5. Novis CA, Rubin ML. Diplopia resolution: perspectives in refraction. Surv Ophthalmol 1995;39:396.
6. Archer SM. Abnormal head posture in patients with third and sixth nerve palsy. Am Orthoptic J1995;45:34.
7. Saunders RA, Roberts EL. Abnormal head posture in patients with fourth cranial nerve palsy. Am Orthoptic J 1995;45:24.
8. von Noorden GK, Campos EC. Binocular Vision and Ocular Motility: Theory and Management of Strabismus, 6th ed. St. Louis: Mosby, 2002.
9. Kushner BJ. Management of diplopia limited to down gaze. Arch Ophthalmol 1995;113:1426.
10 Helveston EM. Surgical Management of Strabismus: An Atlas of Strabismus Surgery, 4th ed. St. Louis: Mosby, 1993.
11. Kerkhoff G, Stogerer E. Recovery of fusional convergence after systematic practice. Brain Inj 1994;8:15.

4

Headaches

OVERVIEW

Treating headaches is much like cooking: We all have our favorite recipe for the same dish. I (RT) will outline my distillation of the literature combined with my personal biases. There are many more treatment options than those listed here, but I have found that many headaches can be managed adequately with just a few standard drugs. Of course, much more is known about headaches than the information given here; the reader is referred to the references and selected readings for more details about the nosology, pathophysiology, and pharmacology of headache treatment.

Remember that successful pharmacotherapy requires adequate doses of medication taken faithfully. For example, just because the patient has taken propanolol (Inderal) in the past for migraines and reports that "it didn't work" does not mean that it cannot be tried again at a higher dose.

The most common types of headache seen in two major headache clinics were migraine and tension-type, accounting for more than 90% of the total diagnoses [1].

MIGRAINE

Migraine comes in many forms, but in my neuro-ophthalmology practice, the three most common subtypes are visual migraine aura (International Headache Society classification [IHS] 1.3.3 migraine aura without headache), visual migraine aura with headache (IHS 1.3.1 migraine with typical aura), and common migraine (IHS 1.1 migraine without aura).* Unfortunately, when it comes to treatment, much more scientific data is available regarding treatments for common migraine than for migraine with visual components. Thus, we are forced to extrapolate to some degree when treating these other entities. See Boxes 4-1 and 4-2 for characteristics of migraine [2].

The approach to migraine treatment is to use abortive treatments (Box 4-3, Table 4-1), prophylactic treatments (Table 4-2), or both.

Abortive Treatments for Migraine

Ergotamine is a standard drug in the treatment of migraine and has been judged safe and effective by the American Academy of Neurology when used in appropriate dosages and when patients with contraindications are excluded [3].

---

*These numbers are from the newly revised classification.

Box 4-1 Characteristics of Migraine Headache

Often is, or begins, hemicranial.
Throbbing or aching in character; moderate-to-severe intensity.
Reaches a crescendo within minutes to hours; lasts 4-72 hours.
Usually accompanied by photophobia and phonophobia; aggravated by movement.
Often associated with autonomic symptoms like anorexia, nausea, vomiting, diaphoresis, nasal congestion, and lacrimation.
May be precipitated by dietary factors such as alcohol, tyramine-rich foods, monosodium glutamate, foods preserved with nitrites, etc., or changes in lifestyle (e.g., lack of sleep, stress).
Affects women about twice as often as men.

Box 4-2 Common Characteristics of Visual Migraine Aura

Perception of movement is almost universal.
Perception of primary colors or silver and black is often reported.
Visual disturbance frequently has a geometric pattern (fortification scotoma).
Visual disturbance begins in a small portion of visual field, expands over 10-20 minutes to involve both visual fields to some extent, and gradually resolves.*

*The exception is retinal migraine.
For interesting discussions, see Critchley M. Aurae and prodromes in migraine. In: The Citadel of the Senses. New York: Raven, 1986;199; and Sacks O. Migraine: Revised and Expanded. Berkeley: University of California Press, 1992;51.

Box 4-3 Popular Abortive Treatments for Migraine

Ergotamine preparations (e.g., Cafergot)
Combination drugs (e.g., Midrin, Fiorinal, Fioricet, Esgic)
Nonsteroidal anti inflammatory drugs (see Table 4-2)
Over-the-counter sinus medications (e.g., Sinutab, Sine-Off)
Triptans (see Table 4-1)

Table 4-1 Triptans for Abortive Treatment of Migraine

Generic name	Brand Name (USA)	Formulations
Sumatriptan succinate	Imitrex	Injection; oral; nasal spray
Rizatriptan benzoate	Maxalt	Oral; rapid dissolving tablet
Naratriptan HCl	Amerge	Oral
Zolmitriptan	Zomig	Oral; rapid-dissolving tablet
Almotriptan	Axert	Oral

Table 4-2 Some Prophylactic Treatments for Migraine

Drug	Example
Beta blockers	Propranolol
Tricyclic agents	Amitriptyline
Calcium channel blockers	Verapamil
Antiepileptics	Valproate sodium
Methysergide	Sansert
Antihistamine	Periactin

Table 4-3   Some Nonsteroidal Anti-Inflammatory Drugs Used for Aborting Migraines[a]

Generic Name	Brand Name	How Supplied (mg)	Maximum Daily Dose (mg)
Naproxen Sodium	Anaprox	220,[b] 275, 550	1,000
Ibuprofen	Motrin	220,[b] 300-800	3,200
Ketoprofen	Orudis	12.5,[b] 25-75	300
Flurbiprofen	Ansaid	50,100	300

[a]Can be used for migraine prophylaxis as well.
[b]Indicates dosage of over-the-counter preparation.

Nonsteroidal anti-inflammatory drugs (NSAIDs) are favored by many headache experts (Table 4-3). Naproxen sodium (Anaprox; Aleve, over-the-counter) is recommended because of its relative safety, efficacy, and lack of dependence development [4,5]. Also, it does not interfere with the antiplatelet effects of aspirin. Naproxen sodium should be taken in a high first dose, at least 750 mg, to be effective for acute migraine treatment. Smaller doses can be repeated if needed.

NSAIDs are sometimes combined with metoclopramide (Reglan, 5-10 mg), which speeds absorption, acts as an antinauseant, and has serotonergic properties. Aspirin, acetaminophen, and dihydroergotamine have also been combined with metoclopramide with good effect [6,7].

Nonprescription preparations marketed for sinus headache often work well in the acute treatment of migraine. Indeed, many patients with migraine think they have sinus problems causing their headaches. Sinus preparations contain an analgesic (aspirin or acetaminophen), a vasoconstrictor (pseudoephedrine or phenylpropanolamine), and sometimes an antihistamine (Chlor-Trimeton). Patients with hypertension should be warned not to take the combinations containing phenylpropanolamine, because this compound raises blood pressure significantly in certain individuals.

The triptans (see Table 4-1) are the "gold standard" for abortive migraine therapy. If one brand of triptan fails, it is worth trying another since there is a variation in response between the different agents [8].

Opiates are not generally first-line drugs for headache treatment because of side effects, tolerance, and the potential for addiction [2].

Migraine Prophylaxis

Patients should be encouraged to avoid precipitating factors, such as ingestion of certain foods or beverages, or alterations in lifestyle [9]. Prophylactic therapy is usually recommended if migraines are disabling, if they occur more than twice a week, or if the patient is using analgesics on a daily basis [10]. Posing the question "If I could give you a medication to take on a daily basis to prevent the headaches, would you take it?" is often useful in assessing potential compliance.

A number of drug classes have been used for migraine prophylaxis (Tables 4-2 and 4-4). The patient should be warned that monotherapy can be expected to reduce the frequency and severity of attacks, possibly

Table 4-4   Tricyclic Agents in Decreasing Order of Sedation

Generic Name	Brand Name	Smallest Dose (mg)	Maximum Daily Dose (mg)
Amitriptyline	Elavil	10	150
Imipramine	Tofranil	10	200
Nortriptyline	Pamelor	10	100
Desipramine	Norpramin	10	200
Protriptyline	Vivactil	5	40

Source: Cada DJ, Covington TR, Hussar DA, et al. Drug Facts and Comparisons, 48th ed. St. Louis: Facts and Comparisons, 1994.

up to 70%, but will probably not be curative [2,10]. First-line, high-efficacy drugs with mild-to-moderate adverse event profile are porpranolol, timolol, amitriptyline, and valproate [2,10]. Patient therapy should be individualized. For example, for a patient with hypertension, a beta-blocker, would be a good first choice whereas a person with a mixture of migraine and tension-type headache would probably benefit from amitriptyline as a first drug of choice [2,10].

Beta blockers and tricyclic agents seem to be equally effective [11], calcium channel blockers less so. Valproate is very effective [10,12]. Other anti-epileptic drugs with promise for migraine prophylaxis are gabapentin (Neurontin) and topiramate (Topamax) [10,12]. Tricyclic agents are often effective more quickly and at lower doses when prescribed for migraine prophylaxis than when prescribed for depression. Small doses are started, with increases every third to seventh day to minimize side effects [5]. Low-dose aspirin alone may be effective in migraine prophylaxis [11,13,14]. Raskin [4] suggests alternating drug classes every month as in ergotamine, beta blocker, and tricyclic in patients with difficult-to-control migraines. The use of botulinum toxin type A (BTX) for migraine prophylaxis is currently being studied [10].

In patients with migraine headache and visual disturbances, I recommend one 325-mg aspirin per day and tend to prescribe calcium channel blockers more often as my first choice for prophylaxis [5,13,15]. Amitriptyline has vasorelaxing properties, making it another reasonable choice. The prohibition of the use of propranolol in patients with visual migraine aura probably has no basis [10].

The treatment of isolated visual migraine aura is problematic unless reassurance alone is adequate. Anecdotal reports exist of positive effects from topirimate, valproate, gabapentin, and angiotensin converting enzyme inhibitors.

TENSION-TYPE HEADACHE (IHS 2.1-2.4)

Tension-type headache is the most common primary headache with a lifetime prevalence of 30-78%. The drug of choice for tension-type headache is a tricyclic antidepressant, with amitriptyline (e.g., Elavil) the most preferred [16]. When writing a tricyclic prescription for headache, I have found it useful to specify "for headache." This obviates the

---

Box 4-4   Some Characteristics of Tension-Type Headache

Steady pain, nonpulsatile (tightness, pressure, "like wearing a hat that's too
  tight"), usually generalized
Mild-to-moderate intensity
Not aggravated by physical activity
No prodrome or aura
Episodic (<15 days/month) or chronic (>15 days/month)
Often associated with depression or anxiety
May have sore-to-touch head, neck, and back muscles
History of multiple doctor visits for headache

Box 4-5   Some Alternative Headache Treatments

Magnesium, 250-400 mg/d
Vitamin B2 (Riboflavin), 400 mg/d
Feverfew (available in health food stores)
Ginger, 500-600 mg mixed with water (anti-inflammatory and antihistamine
  effects)
Fish oil (omega-3 fatty acids)
Biofeedback

---

pharmacist quizzing the patient about his or her "depression,"
subsequent confusion on the part of the patient, and embarrassing
telephone calls to the doctor. The dose of tricyclic agent for headache
therapy tends to be lower than that needed for treating depression. See
Box 4-4 for a list of characteristics of tension-type headache.

ANALGESIC REBOUND HEADACHE (IHS 8.2)

Drug-induced chronic daily headache (medication overuse headache;
"painkiller headache") is caused by frequent use of opioids, analgesics,
ergotamine, or triptans at least twice a week, or more frequently, for at
least 1 month [17]. It may be confused with chronic tension-type
headache unless a careful drug history is obtained. The treatment is
appropriate patient education and a weaning schedule from the
offending agent or agents.

OTHER TREATMENTS FOR HEADACHES

Many patients with headaches are interested in trying holistic or
alternative nonprescription treatments (Box 4-5). Many of these have
scientific merit [10,19].

  The National Headache Foundation and the American Council for
Headache Education have newsletters oriented toward laypersons and
other interested parties [19,20].

REFERENCES
1. Raskin NH. Headache, 2nd ed. New York: Churchill Livingstone, 1988.
2. Goadsby PJ, Lipton RB, Ferrari MD. Migraine—current understanding and
   treatment. N Engl J Med 2002;346:257.

3. Quality Standards Subcommittee of the American Academy of Neurology. Practice parameter: appropriate use of ergotamine tartrate and dihydroergotamine in the treatment of migraine and migraine status (summary statement). Neurology 1995;45:585.

4. Raskin NH. Headache. West J Med 1994;161:299.

5. Daroff RB, Whitney-Rainbolt CM. Treatment of Headaches and Facial Pain. In Tusa RJ, Newman SA (eds): Neuro-Ophthalmological Disorders: Diagnostic Work-up and Management. New York: Marcel Dekker, 1995;621.

6. Gross DW, Donat JR, Boyle CAJ. Dihydroergotamine and metoclopramide in the treatment of organic headaches. Headache 1995;35:637.

7. Daroff RB, Whitney CM. Treatment of vascular headaches. Headache 1986;26:470.

8. Ferrari MD, Goadsby PJ, Roon KI, Lipton RB. Triptans (serotonin, 5-HT 1B/1D agonists) in migraine: detailed results and methods of a meta-analysis of 53 trials. Cephalalgia 2002;22:633.

9. Spierings ELH. Migraine prevention and errors in living: Dr. Graham's lessons for patients and physicians. Headache 2002;42:153.

10. Silberstein SD, Goadsby PJ. Migraine preventive treatment. Cephalalgia 2002;22:491.

11. Cada DJ, Covington TR, Hussar DA, et al. Drug Facts and Comparisons, (48th ed). St. Louis: Facts and Comparisons, 1994.

11. Ziegler DK, Hurwitz A, Preskorn S, et al. Propranolol and amitriptiline in prophylaxis of migraine: pharmacologic and therapeutic effects. Arch Neurol 1993;50:825.

12. Cutrer FM. Antiepileptic drugs: How they work in headache. Headache 2001;41(Suppl 1):S3.

13. Buring JE, Peto R, Hennekens CH. Low-dose aspirin for migraine prophylaxis. JAMA 1990;264:1711.

14. Dalessio DJ. Aspirin prophylaxis for migraine. JAMA 1990;264:1721.

15. Silberstein SD, Young WB. Migraine aura and prodrome. Semin Neurol 1995;15:175.

16. Zagami AS. Chronic tension-type headache: rational drug treatment options. CNS Drugs 1995;4:90.

17. Silberstein SD, Welch KMA. Painkiller headache. Neurology 2002;59:972.

18. Mauskop A, Altura BT, Cracco RQ, et al. Deficiency in serum ionized magnesium but not total magnesium in patients with migraines-possible role of ionized calcium/magnesium ratio. Headache 1993;33:135.

19. National Headache Foundation, 428 West St. James Place, 2nd FL, Chicago, IL 60614-2750. Available at www.headaches.org.

20. American Council for Headache Education, 19 Mantua Rd, Mt. Royal, NJ 08061. Available at www.achenet.org.

SELECTED READINGS

Silberstein SD, Lipton RB, Dalessio DJ (eds). Wolff's Headache and Other Head Pain, 7th ed. New York: Oxford University Press, 2001.

Silberstein SD. Practice parameter: Evidence-based guidelines for migraine headache (an evidence-based review). Report of the Quality Standards Subcommittee of the American Academy of Neurology. Neurology 2000;55:754.

Diamond ML, Solomon GD (eds). Diamond and Dalessio's The Practicing Physician's Approach to Headache, 6th ed. Philadelphia: WB Saunders, 1999.

Olesen J, Tfelt-Hansen P, Welch KMA (eds).The Headaches. New York: Raven, 1993.

5

Low-Tension (or Normal Tension) Glaucoma

OVERVIEW AND ETIOLOGY

Low-tension glaucoma (LTG), also called normal-tension glaucoma (NTG), is a diagnostic and therapeutic conundrum, with the criteria used for defining the condition varying widely [1-3]. This disorder can be broken down into five major categories (Box 5-1). LTG can be mimicked by congenital optic disc anomalies [4] or by acquired optic nerve diseases (Box 5-2) that produce glaucoma-like visual field defects (Box 5-3).

"Burned-out" glaucoma, with glaucomatous optic atrophy and field loss, but with normal pressures, is often seen in cases of pigmentary dispersion [5]. Other subcategories include prior steroid-induced glaucoma and burned-out glaucoma with hyposecretion coupled with a low outflow facility [6]. True glaucoma with wide fluctuations of intraocular pressure is often misdiagnosed as LTG. The diagnosis of multifactorial optic neuropathy, a result of a combination of diseases, requires a very thorough examination of personal and family medical history.* Therefore, true LTG is a diagnosis of exclusion.

In general, LTG is further split into progressive and nonprogressive subtypes. Nonprogressive LTG is usually due to a transient hemodynamic

---

Box 5-1 Categories of Low-Tension Glaucoma
Pseudo-LTG (nonglaucomatous causes for optic atrophy and field loss)
"Burned-out" glaucoma
Atypical glaucoma (wide diurnal fluctuations)
Combination of diseases
True LTG

LTG, Low-tension glaucoma.

---

*J. Lawton Smith said it best: "I'm goin' to tell you my theory for why with a tension of 20 in an eye, the eye goes to pot. I'll tell you why it goes to pot: because the patient has had an old optic nerve contusion, or has a low-grade burned-out uveitis, or has a little bit of some form of genetic optic atrophy, or has some coexisting chiasmal compression, or has had syphilis, etc., etc., etc. What I'm tryin' to tell you is this: you take a little bit of too much tobacco and alcohol, a little bit of sorry diet, grandma who had pernicious anemia, aunt Fat Back who had multiple sclerosis, a big dilated and tortuous carotid siphon bangin' on the chiasm, a blood pressure of 155 over 98, you take all those things, a little tad of uveitis back down the road, maybe funny lookin' discs in the first place and then you add a tension of 20 on that guy and he loses field. I think what's goin' on is that he's got a combination of diseases." (Quoted from JL Smith, Tape #71, The Low-Tension Glaucomas. Miami: Neuro-ophthalmology Tapes, 1976.)

Box 5-2   Differential Diagnosis of Glaucomatous Optic Atrophy

Congenital disc dysplasias
Colobomas
Morning glory disc anomaly
Optic pits

Acquired optic atrophy with cupping
Dominant optic atrophy
Ischemic optic neuropathy (especially due to arteritis)
Optic disc infarction
Compressive optic neuropathies

Source: Shields JA. Textbook of Glaucoma (3rd ed). Baltimore: Williams & Wilkins, 1992;172.

Box 5-3   Anterior Visual Pathway Lesions Causing Glaucoma-Like Visual Field Defects

Generalized depression of the visual field
Functional visual loss
Rod and cone dystrophies
Bilateral occipital lobe infarctions with macular sparing
Chronic atrophic papilledema

Nerve fiber bundle defects
Retinal or chorioretinal lesions
Rod and cone dystrophies
Choroiditis and retinochoroiditis
Branch retinal artery occlusions
Macular ischemia

Nonglaucomatous optic nerve disease
Optic disc dysplasias, especially pits and colobomas
Hereditary optic neuropathies (e.g., dominant optic atrophy, Leber's hereditary
    optic neuropathy)
Ischemic optic neuropathy
Optic neuritis
Chronic papilledema
Compressive optic neuropathies
Toxic and nutritional optic neuropathies

---

catastrophe and, thus, is actually a form of pseudo-LTG [7-10]. Progressive LTG may worsen more rapidly than primary open-angle glaucoma despite medical and surgical treatment [11]. The recent reports of the Collaborative Normal-Tension Glaucoma Study Group emphasize the capricious nature and variability of progression of the disease when untreated [12,13]. Both eyes are affected in approximately 70% of patients, and the disease is more commonly seen in patients older than 60 years of age [14]. Women are affected about twice as often as men, and LTG represents 10-30% of all forms of glaucoma [15].

PATHOGENESIS

As one might expect, vascular etiologies for LTG are most prevalent, with nocturnal hypotension [7,16], sleep apnea [17,18], and vasospasm

Box 5-4   Key Historic Points in the Evaluation of Low-Tension Glaucoma

Any serious operation or accident with significant blood loss
Any episode of sudden vision loss
Cardiac arrest or myocardial infarction
Eye surgery or brain surgery
Migraine
Pernicious anemia
Poor nutrition
Raynaud's phenomenon (and other connective tissue and autoimmune diseases)
Steroids (topical or systemic)
Syphilis
Tobacco or alcohol abuse
Toxins (e.g., ethambutol, methotrexate)
Trauma to eye or head
Uveitis

[19-21] as precipitating factors. The ultimate insult appears to be low ocular perfusion pressure, either transient or chronic [22]. Optic disc blood flow is influenced by the relationship between intraocular pressure and mean systemic pressure. Fluorescein angiography of patients with progressive LTG shows development of new filling defects in the optic disc [23]. Blood flow velocity, as measured by color Doppler imaging, has been reportedly reduced in LTG patients [24-26]. Recent interest in the vasoactive peptide endothelin-1 (ET-1) has led to studies that show increased plasma levels in patients with LTG [27-30]. In rabbits, intravitreal or intravenous injection of ET-1 causes decreased optic nerve and choroidal blood flow [29]. Magnetic resonance imaging (MRI) of the brains of patients with LTG suggests that they have more diffuse small-vessel ischemic changes than healthy control subjects [31]. Optic disc hemorrhages are a negative prognostic factor for visual field loss in patients with LTG [32].

HISTORY

As in many areas of medicine, patient history is extremely important in separating true LTG from imposters. Important historic points are listed in Box 5-4. A family history of glaucoma [33], unexplained transient vision loss, and connective tissue and autoimmune diseases are also important considerations in the diagnosis of true LTG [34].

EXAMINATION

During the office examination special attention should be given to the following areas. Blood pressure should be checked in both arms with the patient supine and erect. A slit-lamp examination should include a search for iris transillumination defects, iris atrophy, and corneal endothelial abnormalities indicative of previous inflammation. Gonioscopy should be performed to look for increased pigmentation in the filtration angles, angle recession, and peripheral anterior synechiae. Intraocular pressures should be measured before and after pupillary dilation, and a diurnal pressure curve should be considered. Retinal artery pressures should be estimated by ophthalmodynamometry or other means. The carotid arteries should be auscultated. The optic discs should be studied carefully and photographed, and special attention should be given to the visual field examination [35].

INVESTIGATIONS

Investigations such as a fluorescent treponemal antibody absorption test for syphilis, carotid artery evaluation, sleep study, and ambulatory blood pressure monitoring may be useful. Magnetic resonance imaging, computed tomography, or both may be appropriate [36].

TREATMENT

From the foregoing it is apparent that the first step when LTG is suspected is to be sure of the diagnosis of true progressive LTG. Thereafter, the traditional approach has been to decrease intraocular pressure to levels low enough to stop progressive vision loss. The Collaborative Normal-Tension Glaucoma Study Group found that lowering intraocular pressure 30%, medically or surgically, had a very significant effect in protecting patients with LTG from glaucomatous disc changes and visual field loss over a 5-year study period [37].

The evidence implicating nocturnal hypotension and vasospasm in the pathogenesis of LTG offers new potential interventions. Hayreh and coworkers [7] caution against vigorous antihypertensive therapy in formerly hypertensive patients with LTG. Common sense dictates daytime dosing in these patients. Flammer [38] has reported the anecdotal use of a fluorinated steroid (fludrocortisone) in systemically hypotensive patients with progressive vision loss. Calcium channel blockers, particularly — but not exclusively — nifedipine, have been proposed to be beneficial in LTG [38-40]. Topical verapamil decreases retinal vascular resistance in humans without ocular disease [41], and an ophthalmic formulation of this drug is under development. In this regard, vasospastic amaurosis fugax has been successfully treated with nifedipine and verapamil [42]. In one study, nimodipine improved contrast sensitivity in patients with LTG [43]. Topical betaxolol, a selective beta-adrenergic blocker, may have vasorelaxant effects in patients with LTG [44,45].

REFERENCES

1. Shields JA. Textbook of Glaucoma (3rd ed). Baltimore: Williams & Wilkins, 1992;172.
2. Chumbley LC, Brubaker RF. Low-tension glaucoma. Am J Ophthalmol 1976;81:761.
3. Lee BL, Bathija R, Weinreb RN. The definition of normal-tension glaucoma. J Glaucoma 1998;7:366.

4. Brodsky MC. Congenital optic disk anomalies. Surv Ophthalmol 1994;39:89.
5. Ritch R. Nonprogressive low-tension glaucoma with pigmentary dispersion. Am J Ophthalmol 1982;94:190.
6. Panek WC, Lee DA, Christensen RE. Low-tension glaucoma. Glaucoma 1989;11:99.
7. Hayreh SS, Zimmerman MB, Podhajsky P, et al. Nocturnal arterial hypotension and its role in optic nerve head and ocular ischemic disorders. Am J Ophthalmol 1994;117:603.
8. Lichter PR, Henderson JW. Optic nerve infarction. Am J Ophthalmol 1978;85:302.
9. Connolly SE, Gordon KB, Horton JC. Salvage of vision after hypotension-induced ischemic optic neuropathy. Am J Ophthalmol 1994;117:235.
10. Kitazawa Y, Shirato S, Yamamoto T. Optic disc hemorrhage in low-tension glaucoma. Ophthalmology 1986;93:853.
11. Gliklich RE, Steinmann WC, Spaeth GL. Visual field change in low-tension glaucoma over a five-year follow-up. Ophthalmology 1989;96:316.
12. Drance S, Anderson DR, Schulzer M, et al. Risk factors for progression of visual field abnormalities in normal-tension glaucoma. Am J Ophthalmol 2001;131:699.
13. Anderson DR, Drance SM, Schulzer M, et al. Natural history of normal tension glaucoma. Ophthalmology 2001;108:247.
14. Drance SM. Low-tension glaucoma. Arch Ophthalmol 1985;103:1131.
15. Kamal D, Hitchings R. Normal tension glaucoma — a practical approach. Br J Ophthalmol 1998;82:835.
16. Graham SL, Drance SM. Nocturnal hypotension: role in glaucoma progression. Surv Ophthalmol 1999;43:Suppl 1:S6.
17. Mojon DS, Hess CW, Goldblum D, et al. High prevalence of glaucoma in patients with sleep apnea syndrome. Ophthalmology 2000;107:816.
18. Marcus DM, Costarides AP, Gokhale P, et al. Sleep disorders: a risk for normal-tension glaucoma? J Glaucoma 2001;10:177.
19. Phelps CD, Corbett JJ. Migraine and low-tension glaucoma. Invest Ophthalmol Vis Sci 1985;26:1105.
20. Corbett JJ, Phelps CD, Eslinger P, et al. The neurologic evaluation of patients with low-tension glaucoma. Invest Ophthalmol Vis Sci 1985;26:1101.
21. Cursiefen C, Wisse M, Cursiefen S, et al. Migraine and tension headache in high-pressure and normal-pressure glaucoma. Am J Ophthalmol 2000;129:102.
22. Schwenn O, Troost R, Vogel A, et al. Ocular pulse amplitude in patients with open angle glaucoma, normal tension glaucoma, and ocular hypertension. Br J Ophthalmol 2002;86;981.
23. Talusan ED, Schwartz B, Wilcox LM. Fluorescein angiography of the optic disc: a longitudinal follow-up study. Arch Ophthalmol 1980;98:1579.
24. Yamazaki Y, Hayamizu F. Comparison of flow velocity of ophthalmic artery between primary open angle glaucoma and normal tension glaucoma. Br J Ophthalmol 1995;79:732.
25. Butt Z, McKillop G, O'Brien C, et al. Measurement of ocular blood flow velocity using colour Doppler imaging in low tension glaucoma. Eye 1995;9:29.
26. Harris A, Sergott RC, Spaeth GL, et al. Color Doppler analysis of ocular vessel blood velocity in normal-tension glaucoma. Am J Ophthalmol 1994;118:642.
27. Kaiser HJ, Flammer J, Wenk M, et al. Endothelin-1 plasma levels in normal-tension glaucoma: abnormal response to postural changes. Graefes Arch Clin Exp Ophthalmol 1995;233:484.
28. Salom JB, Torregrosa G, Alborch E. Endothelins and the cerebral circulation. Cerebrovasc Brain Metab Rev 1995;7:131.
29. Sugiyama T, Moriya S, Oku H, et al. Association of endothelin-1 with normal tension glaucoma:clinical and fundamental studies. Surv Ophthalmol 1995;39(Suppl 1):S49.

30. Haefliger IO, Meyer P, Flammer J, et al. The vascular endothelium as a regulator of the ocular circulation: a new concept in ophthalmology? Surv Ophthalmol 1994;39:123.

31. Ong K, Farinelli A, Billson F, et al. Comparative study of brain magnetic resonance imaging findings in patients with low tension glaucoma control subjects. Ophthalmology 1995;102:1632.

32. Ishida K, Yamamoto T, Sugiyama K, Kitazawa Y. Disk hemorrhage is a significantly negative prognostic factor in normal-tension glaucoma. Am J Ophthalmol 2000;129:707.

33. Bennett SR, Alward WLM, Folberg R. An autosomal dominant form of low-tension glaucoma. Am J Ophthalmol 1989;108:238.

34. Yamamoto T, Maeda M, Sawada A, et al. Prevalence of normal-tension glaucoma and primary open-angle glaucoma in patients with collagen diseases. Jpn J Ophthalmol 1999;43:539.

35. Yoshikawa K, Inoue T, Inoue Y. Normal tension glaucoma: the value of predictive tests. Acta Ophthalmol Scand Suppl 1993;71:463.

36. Gutman I, Melamed S, Ashkenazi I, et al. Optic nerve compression by carotid arteries in low-tension glaucoma. Graefes Arch Clin Exp Ophthalmol 1993;231:12.

37. Anderson DR, Drance SM, Schulzer M, et al. Comparison of glaucomatous progression between untreated patients with normal-tension glaucoma and patients with therapeutically reduced intraocular pressures. Am J Ophthalmol 1998;126:487.

38. Flammer J. Therapeutic aspects of normal-tension glaucoma. Curr Opin Ophthalmol 1993;4:58.

39. Netland PA, Chaturvedi N, Dreyer EB. Calcium channel blockers in the management of low-tension and open-angle glaucoma. Am J Ophthalmol 1993;115:609.

40. Ishida K, Yamamoto T, Kitazawa Y. Clinical factors associated with progression of normal-tension glaucoma. J Glaucoma 1998;7:372.

41. Netland PA, Grosskreutz CL, Feke GT, et al. Color Doppler ultrasound analysis of ocular circulation after topical calcium channel blocker. Am J Ophthalmol 1995;119:694.

42. Winterkorn JMS, Kupersmith MJ, Wirtschafter JD, et al. Brief report: treatment of vasospastic amaurosis fugax with calcium-channel blockers. N Engl J Med 1993;329:396.

43. Bose S, Piltz JR, Breton ME. Nimodipine, a centrally active calcium antagonist, exerts a beneficial effect on contrast sensitivity in patients with normal tension glaucoma and in control subjects. Ophthalmology 1995;102:1236.

44. Harris A, Spaeth GL, Sergott RC, et al. Retrobulbar arterial hemodynamic effects of betaxolol and timolol in normal-tension glaucoma. Am J Ophthalmol 1995;120:168.

45. Hesse RJ. Color Doppler ultrasound measurement of beta-blocker response in normal tension glaucoma. Neuroophthalmology 1995;15:259.

6

Nutritional Deficiency Amblyopia

OVERVIEW

Nutritional deficiency amblyopia (NDA) is a problem seen frequently in neuro-ophthalmology practices, especially if serving patients from a diverse socioeconomic background. In Lessell's practice, the diagnosis of toxic or NDA was made in 7% of patients seen for optic neuropathy or vision failure of uncertain cause [1]. This condition was the fifth most common final diagnosis of a total of 55 diagnoses in his series.

NDA is most commonly seen in malnourished alcoholics [1,2] but is documented in other settings as well (Box 6-1). Victor points out that as of 1979 there were about 10 million alcoholics in the United States; only approximately 3% of these patients suffered from a nutritional deficiency disease affecting the nervous system [2]. This observation leads to a fundamental point on which most experts agree: refined ethanol per se is not toxic to the visual system in the vast majority of cases. Rather, deficiency of essential vitamins and nutrients, especially thiamine (vitamin B_1), cobalamin (vitamin B_{12}), and folic acid is responsible. This has been proven, for example, by the clinical observation that alcoholics with nutritionally associated visual loss who take thiamine supplements and continue to drink immoderately characteristically improve [1-5].

Folate-responsive optic neuropathy has been reported [6]. Six patients who smoked and drank excessively were folate deficient according to blood tests. Vision improved in all within 2 months after folate supplementation only (1 mg per day) with no change in personal habits. Pure "tobacco amblyopia" was reported in two patients — one a cigar smoker, the other a pipe smoker — by Rizzo and Lessell [7]. The former patient improved after vitamin B_{12} supplements and smoking cessation, and the latter after vitamin B_{12} supplementation alone.

Box 6-1   Some Causes of Nutritional Deficiency Amblyopia*

Chronic alcoholism with thiamine deficiency
Vitamin B_{12} deficiency
Folate deficiency
Following jejunoileal bypass for obesity
Ketogenic diet
Tryptophan deficiency

*See also Jarger W, Kafer O, Schmidt H, et al. Bilateral optic atrophy in childhood caused by tryptophan deficiency. Metab Pediatr Syst Ophthalmol 1979;3:167; Thompson RE, Felton JL. Nutritional amblyopia associated with jejunoileal bypass surgery. Ann Ophthalmol 1982;14:848; and Hoyt CS, Billson FA. Optic neuropathy in ketogenic diet. Br J Ophthalmol 1979;63:191.

Interestingly, neither was vitamin B_{12} deficient by laboratory measures. Cobalamin and folate are intimately related in their metabolism and physiologic effects, and it is not surprising that reports of visual loss from "pure" deficiencies of either one are hard to find [8].

The epidemic of optic neuropathy and peripheral neuropathy in Cuba probably was the result of negative interactions between lack of nutritional factors and exposure to environmental toxins [9-11]. For example, risk factors for disease included cigar smoking and a high carbohydrate diet. Protective factors included antioxidants, B vitamins, and animal products [7,12]. Mitochondrial deoxyribonucleic acid (DNA) mutations did not play a role in epidemic Cuban optic neuropathy [13].

Leber's hereditary optic neuropathy (LHON) is a disease in which maternally inherited mitochondrial DNA mutations are a necessary condition for the disease to be phenotypically expressed. However, not every patient who carries LHON mitochondrial gene mutations develops visual loss. Thus, the possibility that exogenous factors play a role in visual loss in those with LHON mutations has been raised. Cullom and associates found mitochondrial DNA mutations (11778 and 3460) associated with LHON in two of 12 patients diagnosed with tobacco-alcohol amblyopia [14]. Neither of these patients improved with appropriate vitamin supplements. We found a similar association in an alcoholic man with bilateral optic neuropathy who was found to carry the 11778 mutation for LHON [15]. It is of interest that, before the advent of mitochondrial DNA analysis, Friesen noted microvascular fundus changes reminiscent of those seen in LHON in five patients with NDA [16]. However, a case-control study of tobacco and alcohol consumption in patients harboring LHON mutations failed to find any negative associations in this regard [17]. But, the role, or lack thereof, of environmental factors in the expression of visual loss in LHON is not yet settled, because more recent reports of LHON associated with antiretroviral therapy [18] and with the use of ephedra alkaloids [19] have appeared.

Based on clinical and experimental evidence, Sadun concludes that NDA, Cuban epidemic optic neuropathy, and LHON all have abnormal mitochondrial oxidative phosphorylation as a common denominator [20].

SITE OF DAMAGE

Victor described the pathology of NDA as preferentially affecting the papillomacular fibers in the optic nerve just behind the globe and progressing toward the central nervous system — the major finding was demyelination [2]. Dropout of macular ganglion cells was also observed, but was thought to be a secondary event. However, Kupersmith and colleagues found no prolongation of visual-evoked potential P100 latencies, as is characteristic of demyelinating optic neuropathies [21]. These findings might be explained by sparing of other portions of the

---

Box 6-2   Clinical Signs and Symptoms of Nutritional Deficiency Amblyopia

Gradual, bilateral, painless, and usually symmetric loss of vision.
Visual acuities no worse than hand movements.
Dyschromatopsia disproportionately worse than visual acuity.
Visual fields show bilateral cecocentral scotomas.
Peripheral fields never seriously involved.
Fundus examination usually normal early.
Recovery after vitamin supplementation is the rule.

Source: Adapted from Lessell S. Toxic and Deficiency Optic Neuropathies. In Smith JL, Glaser JS (eds), Neuro-ophthalmology (Vol VII). Symposium of the University of Miami and the Bascom Palmer Eye Institute. St. Louis: Mosby, 1973;21.

optic nerve as documented by Victor. Leighton and colleagues [22] described electroretinographic b-wave abnormalities before and after treating patients with NDA with vitamin B_{12}. The b-wave abnormalities improved after treatment, and they concluded that bipolar and Mueller cells were affected in NDA.

CLINICAL SIGNS AND SYMPTOMS

Visual fields often have a pseudo-bitemporal appearance (Figure 6-1) [23]. Patients may fail to recognize all of the Ishihara test plates when visual acuity is no worse than 20/60. Box 6-2 contains a complete list of the clinical signs and symptoms of NDA.

DIFFERENTIAL DIAGNOSIS

A differential diagnosis of bilateral cecocentral scotomas is given in Box 6-3.

HISTORY AND EXAMINATION

A personal history for substance abuse, tobacco use, and use of the various agents listed in Table 6-1 should be obtained [24-45]. A careful family history for hereditary vision loss — especially LHON and dominant optic atrophy — is necessary. Emphasis on visual field testing is mandatory.

Box 6-3   Differential Diagnosis of Bilateral Cecocentral Scotomas

Toxic or nutritional amblyopia
Genetic optic neuropathies (e.g., dominant optic atrophy; LHON)
Optic neuritis
Optic pits
Syphilis
Prechiasmal optic nerve compression

Source: Adapted from Shaw HE, Smith JL. Cecocentral Scotomas-Neuro-ophthalmologic Considerations. In Smith JL (ed), Neuro-ophthalmology Focus 1980. New York: Masson, 1979;165.

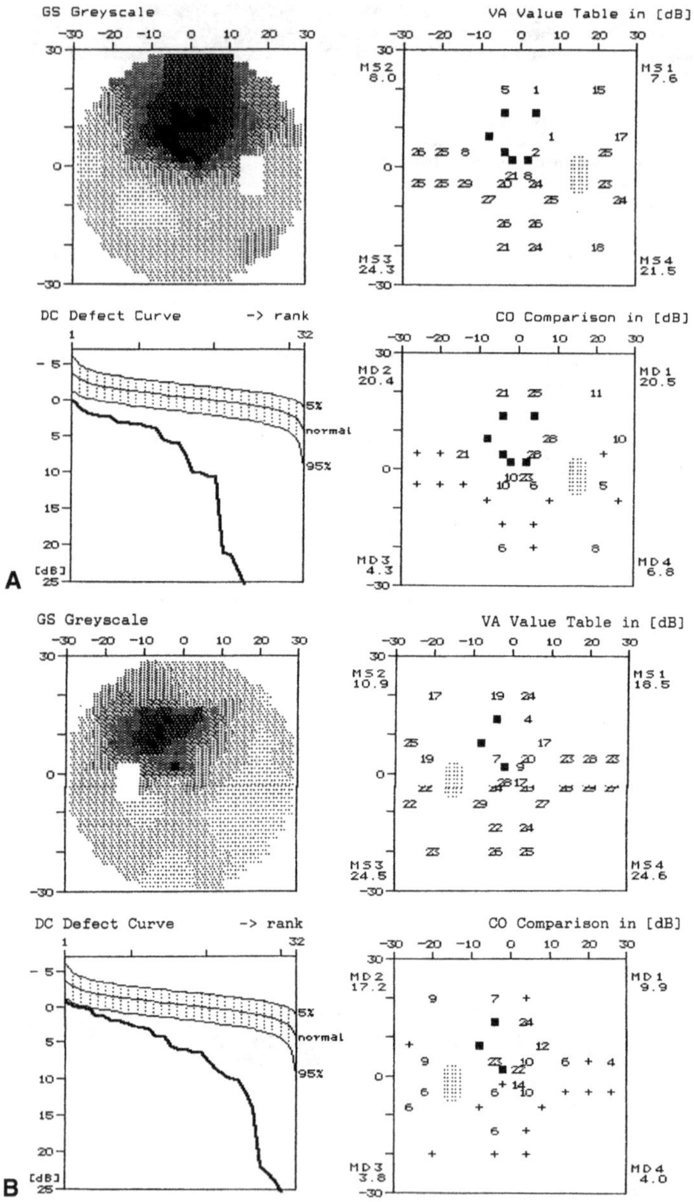

Fig 6-1 Pseudo-bitemporal cecocentral scotomas in a man with nutritional deficiency amblyopia. (Octopus 123 automated perimeter; modified G1X program [Interzeag, Switzerland]). A. Right visual field. B. Left visual field.

Table 6-1 Some Agents Associated with Retina or Optic Nerve Dysfunction	
Agent	Reference
Amiodarone	24
Carbon monoxide	25
Chloramphenicol	26
Chlorpropamide	27
Corticosteroids	28
Digoxin	29
Diiodohydroxyquin	30
Ethambutol	31
Glycine	32
Hexachlorophene	33
Hydroxychloroquine/chloroquine	34
Indomethacin	35
Infliximab	36
Isoniazid	37
Methanol	38
Methotrexate	39
Methyl bromide	40
Niacin	41
Toluene	42
Uremia	43
Vigabatrin	44
Vincristine	45

INVESTIGATIONS

Useful investigations for NDA are listed in Box 6-4. Mitochondrial DNA analysis and contrast-enhanced magnetic resonance imaging should be strongly considered for patients with atypical presentations or in those who do not improve with vitamin supplements.

TREATMENT

Patients with the clinical presentation of NDA are treated with vitamin supplements even if the complete blood cell count and folate and vitamin B_{12} levels are normal. I (RT) recommend one multivitamin with minerals (Centrum or equivalent), one B-100 high-potency B-complex vitamin, and 1-2 mg of folic acid orally each day. B-100 is available generically over the counter (OTC) and contains 100 mg of each of the following: vitamin B_1 (thiamine), vitamin B_2 (riboflavin), niacin,

Box 6-4 Investigations for Nutritional Deficiency Amblyopia
Complete blood cell count, vitamin B_{12}, and folate levels
Venereal Diseases Research Laboratories test, fluorescent treponemal antibody absorption test
Mitochondrial DNA analysis for Leber's hereditary optic neuropathy
Magnetic resonance imaging with contrast enhancement
Screen blood and urine for toxic substances
Test for human immunodeficiency virus

pantothenic acid, and vitamin B_6 (pyridoxine). It also contains 400 µg of folate, and 100 µg of vitamin B_{12} and biotin. A B-50 preparation is also available. I supplement the B-100 with folate, which is available OTC in 400-µg tablets or by prescription, 1-2 mg/day. In my experience, visual function should begin to improve in 4 to 6 weeks. If not, I usually recommend weekly intramuscular vitamin B_{12} injections (1,000 µg) for four weekly doses.

Higher doses of thiamine (up to 5-8 g per day) may be needed [46,47]. There is one report of beneficial effect from zinc sulfate (400 mg per day) on NDA, but I have no experience with use of this regimen [48]. In one patient with vitamin-unresponsive NDA, I tried coenzyme Q_{10} with no beneficial effect [49]. Based on the findings from the Cuban epidemic of optic neuropathy, antioxidant treatment also may be useful for NDA [8].

REFERENCES

1. Lessell S. Toxic and Deficiency Optic Neuropathies. In Smith JL, Glaser JS (eds), Neuro-ophthalmology (Vol VII). Symposium of the University of Miami and the Bascom Palmer Eye Institute. St. Louis: Mosby, 1973;21.
2. Victor M. Neuro-ophthalmic Disorders Due to Alcoholism and Malnutrition. In Smith JL (ed), Neuro-ophthalmology Focus 1980. New York: Masson, 1979;357.
3. Woon C, Tang R, Pardo G. Nutrition and optic nerve disease. Semin Ophthalmol 1995;10:195.
4. Ritter L, Klein R, Klein BE, et al. Alcohol use and age-related maculopathy in the Beaver Dam eye study. Am J Ophthalmol 1995;120:190.
5. Potts AM. Tobacco amblyopia. Surv Ophthalmol 1973;17:313.
6. Golnick KC, Schaible ER. Folate-responsive optic neuropathy. J Neuroophthalmol 1994;14:163.
7. Rizzo JR III, Lessell S. Tobacco amblyopia. Am J Ophthalmol 1993;116:84.
8. Chisholm IA. Serum cobalamin and folate in the optic neuropathy associated with tobacco smoking. Can J Ophthalmol 1978;13:105.
9. Cuba Neuropathy Field Investigation Team. Epidemic optic neuropathy in Cuba: clinical characterization and risk factors. N Engl J Med 1995;333:1176.
10. Sadun AA, Martone JF, Muci-Mendoza R, et al. Epidemic optic neuropathy in Cuba. Eye Findings. Arch Ophthalmol 1994;112:691.
11. Ordunez-Garcia PO, Nieto FJ, Espinosa-Brito AD, Caballero B. Cuban epidemic neuropathy 1991-1994: history repeats itself a century after the "amblyopia of the blockade." Am J Public Health 1996;86:738.
12. Newman NJ. Optic neuropathy. Neurology 1996;46:315.
13. Newman NJ, Torroni A, Brown MD, et al. Epidemic neuropathy in Cuba is not associated with mitochondrial DNA mutations found in Leber's hereditary optic neuropathy patients. Am J Ophthalmol 1994;118:158.
14. Cullom ME, Heher KL, Miller NR, et al. Leber's hereditary optic neuropathy masquerading as tobacco-alcohol amblyopia. Arch Ophthalmol 1993;111:1482.
15. Purohit SS, Tomsak RL. Nutritional deficiency amblyopia or Leber's hereditary optic neuropathy? Neuro-ophthalmology 1997;18:111.
16. Friesen L. Fundus changes in acute malnutritional optic neuropathy. Arch Ophthalmol 1983;101:577.
17. Kerrison JB, Miller NR, Hsu F, et al. A case-control study of tobacco and alcohol consumption in Leber hereditary optic neuropathy. Am J Ophthalmol 2000;130:803.

18. Shaikh S, Ta C, Basham AA, Mansour S. Leber hereditary optic neuropathy associated with antiretroviral therapy for human immunodeficiency virus infection. Am J Ophthalmol 2001;131:143.
19. Warner RB, Lee AG. Leber hereditary optic neuropathy associated with use of ephedra alkaloids. Am J Ophthalmol 2002;134:918.
20. Sadun A. Acquired mitochondrial impairment as a cause of optic nerve disease. Tran Am Ophthalmol Soc 1998;96:881.
21. Kupersmith MJ, Weiss PA, Carr RE. The visual-evoked potential in tobacco-alcohol and nutritional amblyopia. Am J Ophthalmol 1983;95:307.
22. Leighton DA, Bhargava SK, Shail G. Tobacco amblyopia: the effect of treatment on the electroretino-gram. Doc Ophthalmol 1979;46:325.
23. Danesh-Meyer H, Kubis KC, Wolf MA. Chiasmopathy? Surv Ophthalmol 2000;44:329.
24. Feiner LA, Younge BR, Kazmier FJ, et al. Optic neuropathy and amiodarone therapy. Mayo Clin Proc 1987;62:702.
25. Carbon monoxide poisoning causes optic neuropathy. Eye 1998;12:809.
26. Godel V, Nemet P, Lazar M. Chloramphenicol optic neuropathy. Arch Ophthalmol 1980;98:1417.
27. Wymore J, Carter JE. Chlorpropamide-induced optic neuropathy. Arch Intern Med 1982;142:381.
28. Teus MA,Teruel JL, Pascual J, et al. Corticosteroid-induced toxic optic neuropathy. Am J Ophthalmol 1991;112:605.
29. Madreperla SA, Johnson MA, Nakatani K. Electrophysiologic and electroretino-graphic evidence for photoreceptor dysfunction as a toxic effect of digoxin. Arch Ophthalmol 1994;112:807.
30. Pittman FE, Westphal MC. Optic atrophy following treatment with diiodohy-droxyquin. Pediatrics 1974;54:81.
31. Kohler K, Zrenner E, Weiler R. Ethambutol alters spinule-type synaptic connections and induces morphologic alterations in the cone pedicles of the fish retina. Invest Ophthalmol Vis Sci 1995;36:1046.
32. Barletta JP, Fanous MM, Hamed LM. Temporary blindness in the TUR syndrome. J Clin Neuroophthalmol 1994;14:6.
33. Slamovits TL, Burde RM, Klingele TG. Bilateral optic atrophy caused by chronic oral ingestion and topical application of hexachlorophene. Am J Ophthalmol 1980;89:676.
34. Bernstein HN. Ocular safety of hydroxychloroquine sulfate (Plaquenil). South Med J 1992;85:1992.
35. Graham CM, Blach RK. Indomethacin retinopathy. Case report and review. Br J Ophthalmol 1988;72:434.
36. Foroozan R, Buono LM, Sergott RC, Savino PJ. Retrobulbar optic neuritis associated with infliximab. Arch Ophthalmol 2002;120:985.
37. Kass I, Mandel W, Cohen H, et al. Isoniazid as a cause of optic neuritis and atrophy. JAMA 1957;164:1740.
38. Sharpe JA, Hostovsky M, Bilbao JM, et al. Methanol optic neuropathy: a histopathological study. Neurology 1982;32:1093.
39. Johansson BA. Visual field defects during low-dose methorexate therapy. Doc Ophthalmol 1992;79:91.
40. Chavez CT, Hepler RS, Straatsma BR. Methyl bromide optic atrophy. Am J Ophthalmol 1985;99:715.
41. Millay RH, Klein ML, Illingworth DR. Niacin maculopathy. Ophthalmology 1988;95:930.
42. Kiyokawa M. Pattern visual evoked cortical potentials in patients with toxic optic neuropathy caused by toluene abuse. Jpn J Ophthalmol 1999;43:438.

43. Winward KE. Editorial comment: optic neuropathy in uremia. J Clin Neuroophthalmol 1989;9:134.

44. Daneshvar H, Racette L, Coupland SG, et al. Symptomatic and asymptomatic visual loss in patients taking vigabatrin. Ophthalmology 1999;106:1792.

45. Norton SW, Stockman JA 3rd. Unilateral optic neuropathy following vincristine chemotherapy. J Pediatr Ophthalmol Strabismus 1979;16:190.

46. Nichols ME, Meador KJ. Thiamine therapy: a historical perspective (Abstract 715S). Neurology 1993;43:A341.

47. Chataway J, Hardman E. Thiamine in Wernicke's syndrome-how much and how long? Postgrad Med J 1995;71:249.

48. Bechetoille A, Ebran JM, Allain P, et al. Therapeutic effects of zinc sulfate on central scotoma due to optic neuropathy in men exhibiting excessive smoking and drinking habits. J Fr Ophthalmol 1983;6:237.

49. Matthews PM, Ford B, Dandurand RJ, et al. Coenzyme Q10 with multiple vitamins is generally ineffective in treatment of mitochondrial disease. Neurology 1993;43:884.

7

Nystagmus and Oscillopsia Treatment

OVERVIEW

This discussion covers those entities for which treatment data are available: periodic alternating nystagmus (PAN), downbeat and upbeat nystagmus, acquired pendular nystagmus, oculopalatal tremor ("myoclonus"), see-saw nystagmus, saccadic oscillations, superior oblique myokymia, and congenital nystagmus (CN). At the outset, keep in mind that a number of drugs and deficiencies can cause nystagmus and oscillopsia (Table 7-1) [1-5]. From the patient's perspective, the adverse effects of pathologic nystagmus and related eye movement disorders can be twofold: (1) decreased visual acuity or (2) oscillopsia. For example, a patient with CN may have subnormal acuity purely from the CN but will not complain of oscillopsia. By contrast, another individual with acquired pendular nystagmus might be bothered by both oscillopsia and decreased acuity, whereas a third with superior oblique myokymia may complain of intermittent oscillopsia only.

It has been shown that, for detection of objects subtending less than 1 degree of visual space on the retina, retinal slip must be kept under approximately 5 degrees per second. Visual acuity declines in a logarithmic fashion if retinal slip velocity increases above this threshold [6]. In the torsional plane, tolerance for retinal image slip is normally higher [7]. The tolerance for the perception of oscillopsia is more variable [8], but, in cases of acquired nystagmus, oscillopsia is abolished if retinal image drift is reduced to less than 5 degrees per second.

OPTICAL TREATMENTS

Prisms can be used to take advantage of a "null region," if present, in patients with CN. That is, if there is a specific horizontal conjugate gaze angle where the CN is less, base-right or base-left prisms can be used to

Table 7-1 Some Drugs or Deficiencies that Cause Nystagmus or Oscillopsia		
Drug or Deficiency	Type of Nystagmus	Reference
Anticonvulsants	Varied	1
Thiamine deficiency	Gaze-evoked	2
Magnesium deficiency	Downbeat	3
Tobacco	Upbeat	4
Lithium	Downbeat	5

cause a versional movement of the eyes to this new, "quieter" position. One might think of this as a "prismatic" Kestenbaum procedure [9]. Patients in whom CN damps with convergence may benefit from wearing base-out prisms, sometimes with the addition of a minus 1.00 diopter sphere to make up for the stimulation of accommodation by convergence. Sufferers of downbeat nystagmus (DBN) sometimes benefit from symmetric base-down prisms, especially in full-frame reading glasses, to minimize the need for down-gaze, which often aggravates the nystagmus and oscillopsia. A subset of patients with DBN damp their nystagmus through convergence [10].

Another approach uses the combination of high "plus" (i.e., convex, converging) spectacle lenses with high "minus" (i.e., concave, diverging) contact lenses [11]. Image stabilization is best when the converging system focuses the image at the center of rotation of the eye. The diverging contact lens then moves the image into focus on the retina. Because the contact lens moves with the eye, it does not negate the effect of image stabilization produced by the spectacle lens. However, the vestibulo-ocular reflex is disabled as are voluntary eye movements, so this device must be used with the patient stationary. Other problems with this system are common, ranging from problems with contact lens handling because of diminished dexterity from underlying neurologic disease to intolerance to contact lenses.

The wearing of contact lenses sometimes suppresses CN, apparently via stimulation of trigeminal nerve afferent fibers [12].

Recently an electro-optical device has been designed to treat the visual effects of nystagmus. An infrared sensor to monitor eye movements is coupled with a servo-motor device that continuously adjusts Risley prisms. This device seems best suited for persons with acquired pendular nystagmus [13,14].

PHARMACOLOGIC TREATMENTS

The pharmacologic treatments for nystagmus and related eye movements are summarized in Box 7-1. Controlled, masked trials of drug treatments for abnormal eye movements are few in number. Complete discussion of the mechanisms of action of these various agents is beyond the scope of this chapter; see Leigh and Tomsak [15] for further information. However, a few points will be made.

Drug treatments for peripheral vestibular imbalances play a minor role, are used short term (24-48 hours), and are mainly for the symptoms of nausea and vertigo [15].

Gabapentin is often effective in the treatment of acquired pendular nystagmus [16] and superior oblique myokymia [17], but its mechanism of action in these conditions is unknown.

Baclofen, a GABA-b agonist, is very effective in the treatment of periodic alternating nystagmus and, to a lesser extent, for treatment of upbeat and downbeat nystagmus. It is not clear, however, that baclofen works to suppress nystagmus entirely through GABA-ergic mechanisms [18].

Box 7-1   Pharmacologic Treatment of Nystagmus and Related Eye Movements

Vestibular forms of nystagmus
Peripheral imbalance: diphenhydramine, promethazine, prochlorperazine, ondansetron
Central imbalance
    Downbeat nystagmus: clonazepam, baclofen, trihexyphenidyl
    Upbeat nystagmus: baclofen
Central instability
    Periodic alternating nystagmus: baclofen

Nystagmus associated with visual system disorders
See-saw nystagmus: baclofen, clonazepam, ethanol, gabapentin

Nystagmus from disorders of gaze-holding
Acquired pendular nystagmus
In association with disorders of central myelin: gabapentin, memantine, clonazepam, trihexyphenidyl, scopolamine, ethanol, cannabis
As part of oculopalatal tremor ("myoclonus"): gabapentin, valproate, trihexyphenidyl

Saccadic intrusions and oscillation
Square-wave jerks: methylphenidate
Opsoclonus and ocular flutter: clonazepam, propranolol, gabapentin, corticosteroids, intravenous immunoglobulin, plasma exchange

Miscellaneous abnormal eye movements
Superior oblique myokymia: gabapentin, carbamazepine, propranolol
Ocular neuromyotonia: carbamazepine

Data from Leigh RJ, Tomsak RL. Drug treatments for eye movement disorders. J Neurol Neurosurg Psychiatry 2003;74:1.

Botulinum Toxin A

Botulinum toxin A (BTX) injection into selected eye muscles [19,20] or into the retrobulbar space [21-23] has been used with variable results. Leigh and coworkers injected the horizontal rectus muscles of the right eyes of two patients with acquired nystagmus and recorded the results with the scleral search coil technique [19]. The treatment effectively abolished the horizontal component of the nystagmus in the injected eyes of both patients for approximately 2 months. However, side effects including diplopia, ptosis, and worsening of the oscillopsia and vision in the eye not injected limited the effectiveness of the treatment.

A similar study was done by injecting BTX into the retrobulbar space of three patients with acquired pendular nystagmus [23]. A dose-dependent inhibition of nystagmus was found, but side effects including ptosis, diplopia, and filamentary keratitis made the treatment unsatisfactory. Repka and coworkers [24] and Helveston and Pogrebniak [21] have had better results with retrobulbar BTX. All in all, it appears that careful patient selection and an awareness of the potential complications are required for success using this technique.

SURGICAL TREATMENTS

Surgical techniques for congenital nystagmus are designed to increase foveation time, either by turning the eyes to a null position, by decreasing the amplitude of the nystagmus by large horizontal muscle recessions, or by procedures designed to stimulate convergence and thus nystagmus damping [9,12,25-28].

With the exception of superior oblique myokymia (SOM), acquired nystagmus or other related oscillations have not been routinely treated by eye muscle surgery. Weakening procedures on the superior oblique tendon and inferior oblique muscle do abolish SOM and subjective oscillopsia in the majority of cases [29,30].

A promising new surgical technique for treating CN has been pioneered by Dell'Osso and colleagues [12,31,32]. This involves tenotomizing muscles in the appropriate plane of movement without altering the muscle position on the eye. For example, for a patient with predominantly horizontal CN, the four horizontal recti would be tenotomized. This procedure has been shown to damp nystagmus over a broad range of gaze and to increase acuity by favorably altering foveation periods. It is hypothesized that alteration of proprioceptive feedback loops, and possibly other control pathways, is effected by this surgery [12]. Whether or not tenotomy has salutary effects on acquired nystagmus remains to be seen.

SUMMARY

Optical, surgical, and oral pharmacologic treatments for abnormal eye movements may be effective in selected individuals and for selected conditions (e.g., PAN, superior oblique myokymia, CN). However, the results are far from uniformly effective.

REFERENCES

1. Remler BF, Leigh RJ, Osorio I, et al. The characteristics and mechanisms of paroxysmal visual disturbance associated with anticonvulsant therapy. Neurology 1990;40:791.
2. Cogan DG, Witt ED, Goldman-Rakic PS. Ocular signs in thiamine-deficient monkeys and in Wernicke's disease in humans. Arch Ophthalmol 1985;103:1212.
3. Saul RF, Selhorst JB. Downbeat nystagmus with magnesium depletion. Arch Neurol 1981;38:650.
4. Sibony PA, Evinger C, Manning KA. Tobacco-induced primary-position upbeat nystagmus. Ann Neurol 1987;21:53.
5. Monteiro MLR, Sampaio CM. Lithium-induced downbeat nystagmus in a patient with Arnold-Chiari malformation. Am J Ophthalmol 1993;116:648.
6. Demer JL, Amajadi F. Dynamic visual acuity of normal subjects during vertical optotype and head motion. Invest Ophthalmol Vis Sci 1993;34:1894.
7. Ott D, Seidman SH, Leigh RJ. The stability of human eye orientation during visual fixation. Neurosci Lett 1992;142:183.
8. Leigh RJ, Averbuch-Heller L, Tomsak RL, et al. Treatment of abnormal eye movements that impair vision: strategies based on current concepts of physiology and pharmacology. Ann Neurol 1994;36:129.
9. Kestenbaum A. Clinical Methods of Neuro-Ophthalmologic Examination (2nd ed). New York: Grune & Stratton, 1961;396.
10. Lavin PJM, Traccis S, Dell'Osso LF, et al. Downbeat nystagmus with a pseudocycloid waveform: improvement with base out prisms. Ann Neurol 1983;13:621.

11. Yanigloss SS, Stahl JS, Leigh RJ. Evaluation of current optical methods for treating the visual consequences of nystagmus. Ann NY Acad Sci 2002;956:598.
12. Dell'Osso LF. Development of new treatments for congenital nystagmus. Ann NY Acad Sci 2002;956:361.
13. Stahl JS, Lehmkuhle M, Wu K, et al. Prospects for treating acquired pendular nystagmus with servo-controlled optics. Invest Ophthalmol Vis Sci 2000;41:1084.
14. Yanigloss SS, Leigh RJ. Refinement of an optical device that stabilizes vision in patients with nystagmus. Optom Vis Sci 1992;69:447.
15. Leigh RJ, Tomsak RL. Drug treatments for eye movement disorders. J Neurol Neurosurg Psychiatry 2003;74:1.
16. Averbuch-Heller L, Tusa RJ, Fuhry L, et al. A double-blind controlled study of gabapentin and baclofen as treatment for acquired nystagmus. Ann Neurol 1997;41:818.
17. Tomsak RL, Kosmorsky GS, Leigh RJ. Gabapentin attenuates superior oblique myokymia. Am J Ophthalmol 2002;133:721.
18. Buttner U. Drug therapy of nystagmus and saccadic oscillations. Adv Otorhinolaryngol 1999;55:195.
19. Leigh RJ, Tomsak RL, Grant MP, et al. Effectiveness of botulinum toxin administered to abolish acquired nystagmus. Ann Neurol 1992;32:633.
20. Liu C, Gresty M, Lee J. Management of symptomatic latent nystagmus. Eye 1993;7:550.
21. Helveston EM, Pogrebniak AE. Treatment of acquired nystagmus with botulinum A toxin. Am J Ophthalmol 1988;106:584.
22. Ruben ST, Lee JP, O'Neill DO, et al. The use of botulinum toxin for treatment of acquired nystagmus and oscillopsia. Ophthalmology 1994;101:783.
23. Tomsak RL, Remler BF, Averbuch-Heller L, et al. Unsatisfactory treatment of acquired nystagmus with retrobulbar injection of botulinum toxin. Am J Ophthalmol 1995;119:489.
24. Repka MX, Savino PJ, Reinecke RD. Treatment of acquired nystagmus with botulinum neurotoxin. Arch Ophthalmol 1994;112:1320.
25. Anderson JR. Causes and treatment of congenital eccentric nystagmus. Br J Ophthalmol 1953;37:267.
26. Dell'Osso LF, Flynn JT. Congenital nystagmus surgery: a quantitative evaluation of the effects. Arch Ophthalmol 1979;97:462.
27. Helveston EM, Sprunger DT. Strabismus and nystagmus surgery. Curr Opin Ophthalmol 1991;2:702.
28. Zubcov AA, Stark N, Weber A, et al. Improvement of visual acuity after surgery for nystagmus. Ophthalmology 1993;100:1488.
29. de Sa LC, Good WV, Hoyt CS. Surgical management of myokymia of the superior oblique muscle. Am J Ophthalmol 1992;114:693.
30. Brazis PW, Miller NR, Henderer JD, et al. The natural history and results of treatment of superior oblique myokymia. Arch Ophthalmol 1994;112:1063.
31. Hertle RW, Dell'Osso LF, Fitzgibbon EJ et al. Horizontal rectus tenotomy in the treatment of congenital nystagmus (CN): results of a study in ten adult patients (Phase I). Invest Ophthalmol Vis Sci 2001;42:S319.
32. Dell'Osso LF, Hertle RW. Effects of extraocular muscle tenotomy on congenital nystagmus in macaque monkeys. J AAPOS 2002;6:334.

GENERAL REFERENCE

Leigh RJ, Zee DS. The Neurology of Eye Movements, 3rd ed. New York: Oxford University Press, 1999.

8

Ocular Myasthenia

OVERVIEW AND ETIOLOGY

Ocular myasthenia (OM) most commonly presents as diplopia, ptosis, or both, that is variable and characteristically worse toward the end of the day. Like its generalized variant, myasthenia gravis (MG), OM results from dysfunction of the neuromuscular junction caused by autoimmune attack [1]. Serum antibodies to acetylcholine (ACh) receptors are detectable in about 90% of patients with generalized myasthenia but in only about 50% of those with pure ocular involvement [2]. "Seronegative" patients with generalized MG may actually have a different antigenic target: muscle-specific kinase (MuSK) [3]. However, "seronegative" patients with OM do not appear to have MuSK as the antigenic target [4]. OM can mimic any acquired non-rhythmic eye movement disorder with normal pupils. Eye signs occur in up to 90% of patients with MG at presentation, and eye signs only are present in 15-59% of patients [5]. The physiologic and structural features of extraocular muscles seem to predispose the muscles to involvement in MG [1,6,7].

MG presenting with eye signs, if destined to generalize, usually does so within the first 6 months and less commonly after 2 years. The spread from OM to MG is variable depending on the series but an estimate of approximately two thirds is reasonable [4]. Spread is less likely if single-fiber electromyography results are negative [4]. Spontaneous remission occurs in approximately 10% of patients with OM, usually within the first year. Neonatal forms of MG occur in 10-15% of children born to mothers with MG, because of placental transfer of maternal ACh-receptor antibodies. Approximately 10% of all myasthenia occurs in children and young adults, and it is more prevalent in females. In some cases drugs can cause or worsen the signs and symptoms of MG (Box 8-1).

HISTORY AND EXAMINATION

Myasthenic symptoms and signs are variable and tend to worsen with fatigue and stress. No other neuro-ophthalmologic disease has more signs associated with it; a selection of these is presented in Box 8-2. Remember that OM can mimic almost any eye movement disorder.

Lid fatigue on prolonged up-gaze (Figure 8-1) is perhaps the most frequently elicited sign. When testing for lid fatigue, the patient is asked to look up without blinking at the examiner's hand for 1-2 minutes.

Box 8-1   Adverse Effect of Drugs on Myasthenia

Drug-induced myasthenic syndrome
  ᴅ-penicillamine
Aggravating/unmasking agents
  Antibiotics (e.g., aminoglycosides, tetracyclines)
  Cardiovascular drugs (e.g., procainamide, propranolol, quinidine)
  Psychotropic drugs (e.g., lithium, chlorpromazine, cocaine)
  Anticonvulsants (e.g., phenytoin)
  Ocular hypotensives (e.g., timolol [Timoptic])
  Hormonal agents (e.g., corticotropin, corticosteroids, thyroid hormones)
  Others (e.g., acetylcholinesterase inhibitors, methoxyflurane, chloroquine,
    quinine water)

Sources: Argov Z, Mastaglia FL. Disorders of neuromuscular transmission caused by drugs. N Engl J Med 1979;301:409; Daras M, Samkoff LM, Koppel BS. Exacerbation of myasthenia gravis associated with cocaine use. Neurology 1996;46:271; and Verkijk A. Worsening of myasthenia gravis with timolol maleate eyedrops. Ann Neurol 1985;17:211.

Box 8-2   Miscellaneous Eye Signs and Symptoms in Ocular Myasthenia

Lid fatigue on prolonged up-gaze (Figure 8-1)
Enhanced ptosis
Orbicularis oculi weakness
Absent Bell's phenomenon
"Peek" sign
Myasthenic lid twitch (Cogan)
Lid retraction contralateral to myasthenic ptosis
Lid flutter after blinking
Pseudointernuclear ophthalmoplegia
Saccadic abnormalities
  Hypometric large saccades
  Hypermetric small saccades
  Quiver movements
  Hyperfast saccades
  After edrophonium:
    Saccadic hypermetria
    Macrosaccadic oscillations

Sources: Goodwin JA. Ocular manifestations of myasthenia gravis. Ophthalmol Clin North Am 1992;5:495; Weinberg DA, Lesser RL, Vollmer TL. Ocular myasthenia: a protean disorder. Surv Ophthalmol 1994;39:169; Schmidt D. Signs in ocular myasthenia and pseudomyasthenia: differential diagnostic criteria. Neuroophthalmology 1995;15:21; and Leigh RJ, Zee DS. The Neurology of Eye Movements (Vol 2). Philadelphia: FA Davis, 1991;338.

Orbicularis oculi weakness is tested for by attempting to overcome forced lid closure. The presence or absence of Bell's phenomenon should be noted as well.

The "peek" sign is seen in myasthenics in whom, when asked to close the lids gently, one or both inadvertently open slightly or "peek."

Cogan [8] is credited with describing the myasthenic lid-twitch sign. After prolonged down-gaze, refixation to primary position results in overshooting of the upper lid.

Myasthenic ptosis, when unilateral, is often associated with contralateral lid retraction due to Hering's law. Thus, the relatively

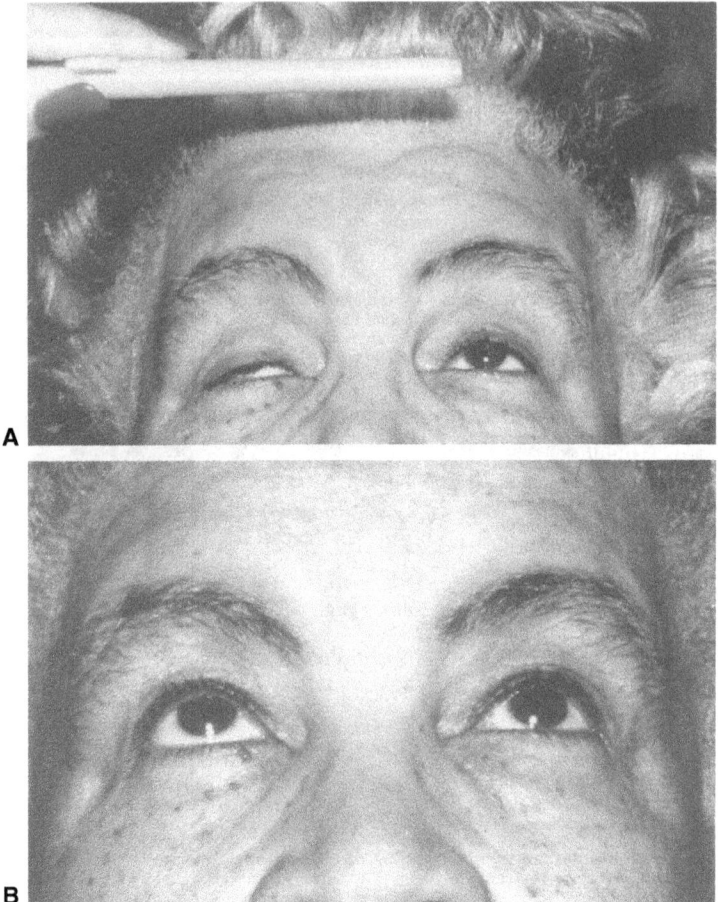

Fig 8-1 A, Myasthenic lid fatigue on prolonged up-gaze. B, Ptosis resolved by intravenous edrophonium injection.

normal lid receives more innervation than necessary in response to attempted elevation of the ptotic lid. Remember that patients with myasthenia may have coincident thyroid eye disease, and this can be a cause for lid retraction as well. "Enhanced ptosis" has also been described wherein lifting the less ptotic lid leads to more ptosis of fellow lid [9].

Internuclear ophthalmoplegia and almost every form of ophthalmoparesis have been simulated by OM. Paradoxically, although versions and ductions are often subnormal in amplitude, the velocity of saccades is often supernormal in MG. This apparently results from differential involvement of the tonic and fast-twitch eye muscle fibers [10].

Box 8-3   Diagnostic Studies for Ocular Myasthenia

Anticholinesterase drugs
  Intravenous edrophonium (Tensilon)
  Intramuscular neostigmine bromide (Prostigmin)
  Oral pyridostigmine (Mestinon)
  Acetylcholine-receptor antibodies
Electromyography
  Repetitive stimulation
  Single fiber
Eye movement recordings before and after edrophonium
Sleep test (improvement in eye signs after sleep or rest)
Ice pack test (improvement in ptosis after cooling lid)

Box 8-4   Other Diagnostic Studies for Ocular Myasthenia

Glucose tolerance test
Skin test for tuberculosis
Antinuclear antibodies
Thyroid function tests
Imaging of mediastinum for thymoma
Antistriated muscle antibodies

Source: Modified from Daroff RB. Ocular Myasthenia: Diagnosis and Therapy. In Glaser JS (ed),
Neuro-ophthalmology: In Memory of Dr. Frank B. Walsh (Vol X). St. Louis: Mosby, 1980;62.

INVESTIGATIONS

Boxes 8-3 and 8-4 summarize investigations for OM.

Intravenous (IV) injection of edrophonium (Tensilon) is the "gold standard" for diagnosing OM. Daroff [5] emphasizes that one needs to demonstrate improvement in function in at least one weak muscle for the Tensilon test (edrophonium test) to be considered positive. Others think that a perverse response (e.g., an esotropia of 15 Δ worsening to an esotropia of 30 Δ) or a paradoxic response (e.g., a right hypertropia becoming a left hypertropia) are positive results.

My (RT) preferred method of performing the Tensilon test is to first ascertain that there is a good sign to observe, preferably ptosis or obvious ophthalmoplegia. Second, I describe the effect to the patient, noting that the onset begins 30-60 seconds after injection and lasts for 1-3 minutes. Lacrimation, salivation, and abdominal cramps are mentioned as common minor side effects and the patient is reassured that the effect will rapidly wear off. Two tenths of 1 cc of edrophonium (10 mg/cc) are injected into a vein in the back of the hand using a 3-cc syringe and a 25-gauge, ⅝-inch needle. If no effect is seen within 30-60 seconds, increments of 1 mg are injected. Most positive responses are seen with Tensilon doses of 4 mg or less [9]. Photographs are taken before and after injection, and eye alignment measures are also documented before and after, if appropriate.

Some recommend the use of an IV butterfly line with atropine handy in case vasovagal side effects occur.

Intramuscular neostigmine (Prostigmin, 0.04 mg/kg mixed with atropine sulfate for body weight) is useful in children. The effect takes approximately 15 minutes to peak and lasts for approximately 30 minutes.

Box 8-5   Some Immunologic Diseases Associated with Ocular Myasthenia

Grave's disease
Hashimoto's thyroiditis
Rheumatoid arthritis
Pernicious anemia
Hemolytic anemia
Systemic lupus erythematosus
Sarcoidosis
Raynaud's syndrome
T-cell lymphoma
Thymoma
Crohn's disease
Acquired immunodeficiency syndrome

Source: Schmidt D. Signs in ocular myasthenia and pseudomyasthenia: differential diagnostic criteria. Neuroophthalmology 1995;15:21.

Occasionally, I prescribe pyridostigmine (Mestinon, 30-60 mg every 2-4 hours while awake) as a therapeutic trial and ask the patient to keep a diary of his or her symptoms in relation to the medication dosage schedule.

The "ice test" has proven useful for diagnosis of OM [4,11]. Here an ice bag is placed on the ptotic eye (or both eyes if ophthalmoparesis is present) and the effect is measured after 5 minutes. One case of anaphylaxis caused by the use of a latex glove to hold the ice has occurred [Daroff, RB. Personal communication.].

ACh-receptor antibodies (binding) are drawn because their presence is virtually diagnostic for MG [2]. As noted previously, circulating ACh-receptor antibodies are detected in approximately 50% of patients with OM, so their absence does not rule out the disease.

Electromyography is elected and performed by neurologists when indicated.

If eye movement recordings can be reliably performed they are useful in the diagnosis of OM, especially if done before and after edrophonium administration [10].

A glucose tolerance test and skin tests for tuberculosis are useful if corticosteroids are considered for treatment. Antinuclear antibodies and thyroid function tests are used to screen for other immunologic diseases associated with MG [12] (Box 8-5).

Imaging the chest with computed tomography or magnetic resonance imaging and screening for antistriated muscle antibodies and antititin antibodies can be considered in patients older than 40 years of age to exclude the presence of thymoma [13].

DIFFERENTIAL DIAGNOSIS

See Box 8-6 for the differential diagnosis of OM. Remember that positive Tensilon test results have been described in patients with brain tumor and ophthalmoplegia, ptosis, or both.

Box 8-6   Differential Diagnosis of Ocular Myasthenia

Fisher's syndrome (ataxia, ophthalmoplegia, and areflexia)
Wernicke's disease
Isolated or combined third, fourth, sixth, or seventh cranial nerve palsies
Brainstem strokes with disorders of gaze
Decompensated strabismus
Spasm of near reflex
Thyroid eye disease
Cerebral/parasellar tumors
Eaton-Lambert myasthenic syndrome
Botulism
Chronic progressive external ophthalmoplegia
Myotonic dystrophy

TREATMENT

My first principle of treatment is to enlist the help of a neurologist in treating patients with OM. As noted previously, OM can generalize to MG. Also, use of some of the treatments listed below are beyond the scope of an ophthalmologist's expertise.

Optical, Mechanical, and Surgical Treatments

Because of the variability of signs and symptoms, optical, mechanical, or surgical treatments for OM are often less effective than for more stable diplopia problems. Occlusion of one eye is a sure cure for binocular diplopia but also restricts the individual to monocular viewing (see Chapter 3). Fresnel prisms are always worth a try if the ocular deviation is stable for weeks. Eye muscle surgery is generally reserved for patients in whom both eyes are severely plegic and awkwardly deviated and signs are stable for at least 5 months [14].

The use of a ptosis "crutch" for ptosis can be helpful, but it is sometimes hard to find an optician who will fashion these correctly. Some patients do well taping their lids partially open for periods of time. In those with severe, bilateral, and unremitting ptosis, some form of reversible lid surgery, such as a frontalis sling, is often useful [15]. Here the surgeon must open the lids just far enough for sight, but not far enough that chronic corneal exposure becomes a problem. If corneal exposure becomes a problem, the procedure can be easily reversed.

Pharmacologic and Immunologic Treatments

Treatments of OM are summarized in Box 8-7.

Mestinon alone rarely alleviates all the symptoms of OM, although it is worth trying. I begin with 30 mg orally (i.e., one half of a 60-mg tablet) every 2-4 hours and ask the patient to keep a log of improvement in symptoms and side effects. If the patient tolerates the medication and improves symptomatically, I increase the dose to 60 mg orally every 2-4 hours while awake. If gastrointestinal side effects occur, I add glycopyrrolate (Robinul), a locally acting anticholinergic, 1-2 mg, orally three times a day. One must always be aware of the possibility of

---

Box 8-7   Treatments for Ocular Myasthenia

Optical/mechanical treatments
   Monocular occlusion for diplopia
   Fresnel prism for diplopia
   Ptosis crutch for ptosis
Medical treatments
   Pyridostigmine (Mestinon)
   Corticosteroids (prednisone)
   Immunosuppressives
     Azathioprine (Imuran)
     Cyclosporine
   Plasmapheresis
   Intravenous gamma globulin
Surgical treatments
   Eye muscle surgery for diplopia
   Eye lid surgery for ptosis
   Thymectomy

---

cholinergic crisis if too much pyridostigmine is given. Therefore, the patient should be told to stop the medication if bulbar symptoms or generalized weakness occurs. A slow-release form of pyridostigmine (Mestinon Timespan, 180 mg) is available but is, in my experience, not very useful for OM. Pyridostigmine is also available as a syrup (Mestinon Syrup, 60 mg/5 ml).

Corticosteroids (e.g., prednisone), with or without pyridostigmine, are sometimes used for the treatment of OM but generally only if the foregoing treatments fail or are unacceptable to the patient. Approximately 90% of patients with MG improve with steroid treatment but the effect takes weeks — even up to a year or more — to reach maximum benefit [2]. Daroff [5] recommends an outpatient dosage schedule beginning with 10 mg of prednisone every other day with increases of 10 mg per day every third dose until symptoms improve or until a maximum of 100 mg every other day is reached. The patient is maintained on the effective dose for 2-3 months before attempting to taper the medication. A slow taper of 10 mg every month is recommended until the dose is reduced to 30 mg every other day. Further decrements are done in 5-mg units until 20 mg is given every day, and then in 2.5-mg increments thereafter. The possibility of relapse or unmasking generalized MG is kept in mind at low doses of prednisone [16].

Kupersmith [17] and Agius [18] advocate the use of daily prednisone at the onset of diagnosis of OM to cause rapid remission and also to possibly prevent generalization. This approach is controversial at present [4,19].

Azathioprine (Imuran) is also effective for MG. It is usually used to spare the side effects of steroids. As with corticosteroids, the beneficial effects may take months to develop. The usual dose is 2-3mg/kg/day [2]. Cyclosporine A, plasmapheresis, mycophenolate, and IV gamma globulin have also been used for generalized MG but are not routinely recommended for ocular signs and symptoms alone [2].

Thymectomy is very effective for OM but rarely prescribed. Approximately 75% of patients with MG have thymic abnormalities, 65% with thymic hyperplasia and 10% with thymoma. Thymoma is rare in patients younger than 40 years of age. The results of thymectomy for generalized MG are very favorable, with about 35% entering complete remission and 50% improving. Although generally not used for OM, thymectomy appears to be at least as successful for pure ocular as for generalized MG [2].

REFERENCES

1. Ubogu EE, Kaminski HJ. The preferential involvement of extraocular muscles by myasthenia gravis. Neuro-ophthalmology 2001;25:219.
2. Drachman DB. Management of ocular myasthenia gravis. In Tusa RJ, Newman SA (eds), Neuro-Ophthalmological Disorders: Diagnostic Work-up and Management. New York: Marcel Dekker, 1995;265.
3. Abicht A, Lochmuller H. What's in the serum of seronegative MG and LEMS? MuSK et al. Neurology 2002;59:1672.
4. Daroff RB. Ocular Myasthenia. In Kaminski HJ (ed), Myasthenia Gravis and Related Diseases. Totowa, NJ: Humana Press, 2003;115.
5. Daroff RB. Ocular myasthenia: diagnosis and therapy. In Glaser JS (ed), Neuro-Ophthalmology: In Memory of Dr. Frank B. Walsh (Vol X). St. Louis: Mosby, 1980;62.
6. Kaminski HJ, Maas E, Spiegel P, et al. Why are eye muscles frequently involved in myasthenia gravis? Neurology 1990;40:1663.
7. Porter JD, Baker RS. Muscles of a different "color": The unusual properties of the extraocular muscles may predispose or protect them in neurogenic and myogenic disease. Neurology 1996;46:30.
8. Cogan DG. Myasthenia gravis: a review of the disease and a description of lid twitch as a characteristic sign. Arch Ophthalmol 1965;74:217.
9. Kupersmith MJ, Latkany R, Straga J. Ocular myasthenia gravis: steroids, Edrophonium dose, thymoma, and generalization. Neuro-Ophthalmol 2001;25:39.
10. Leigh RJ, Zee DS. The Neurology of Eye Movements (Vol 2). Philadelphia: FA Davis, 1991;338.
11. Ellis FD, Hoyt CS, Ellis FJ, et al. Extraocular muscle responses to orbital cooling (ice test) for ocular myasthenia gravis diagnosis. J AAPOS 2000;4:271.
12. Jacobson DM. Acetylcholine receptor antibodies in patients with Graves' Ophthalmopathy. J Neuroophthalmol 1995;15:166.
13. Aarli JA. Titin, thymoma, and myasthenia gravis. Arch Neurol 2001;58:869.
14. Davidson JL, Rosenbaum AL, McCall LC. Strabismus surgery in patients with myasthenia. J Pediatr Ophthalmol Strabismus 1993;30:292.
15. Levine MR. Manual of Oculoplastic Surgery (3rd ed). Philadelphia: Butterworth-Heinemann, 2003;107.
16. Miano MA, Bosely TM, Heiman-Patterson TD, et al. Factors influencing outcome of prednisone dose reduction in myasthenia gravis. Neurology 1991;41:919.
17. Kupersmith MJ, Moster M, Bhiyan S, et al. Beneficial effects of corticosteroids on ocular myasthenia gravis. Arch Neurol 1996;53:802.
18. Agius MA. Treatment of ocular myasthenia with corticosteroids. Arch Neurol 2000;57:750.
19. Kaminski HJ, Daroff RB. Treatment of ocular myasthenia. Arch Neurol 2000;57:752.

9

Optic Glioma

OVERVIEW

Optic nerve gliomas (ONGs), although representing only 1.5-3.5% of all orbital tumors, account for 66% of primary optic nerve tumors [1]. Approximately 25% involve the optic nerve alone, whereas 75% extend to the optic chiasm and/or hypothalamus (OCH). Over 90% of ONGs present within the first two decades; the mean age of presentation is $8\frac{1}{2}$ years [1]. There is a definite relationship between ONG/OCH and neurofibromatosis type 1 (NF-1): 10-70% of patients with ONG involving the OCH (ONG/OCH) have NF-1 (29% is the best estimate) [1]. Bilateral ONGs are almost pathognomonic for NF-1. Also, chiasmal-only involvement is almost never seen in those with NF-1. Patients with NF-1 and ONG/OCH seem to have a more benign course than those without NF-1 [1-5]. For example, mortality in ONG/OCH patients with NF-1 is approximately 50% less than in those not affected with NF-1. Mortality figures double when the chiasm is involved [1]. Mapstone [2] mentions a 60% 10-year survival rate for patients with OCH. The mortality rate in patients with pure ONG is less than 5%, treated or not [1].

Most ONG/OCHs are of the benign pilocytic variety. These are distinctly different from the malignant and universally fatal anterior visual pathway tumors seen in adults [1].

On occasion, meningeal seeding occurs [2,6], and malignant transformation has been reported rarely, especially after radiation therapy [1,7,8] (see Case Study).

Table 9-1   Clinical Signs and Symptoms of Optic Nerve Gliomas at Time of Presentation

Vision loss	85%
Loss of visual field	50%
Optic atrophy	60%
Optic disc edema	50%
Proptosis	95%
Limitation of ocular motility	30%
Nystagmus	24%
Hypothalamic signs	26%
Hydrocephalus	27%

Source: Dutton JJ. Gliomas of the anterior visual pathways. Surv Ophthalmol 1994;38:427.

CLINICAL SIGNS AND SYMPTOMS

ONGs have a characteristically short course of growth followed by stability, slow progression, or regression [3,9,10]. Wilson [9] points out that unilateral ONG rarely invades the central nervous system, and death from this extension is extremely rare. Vision stability is common for up to 6 years [1] but does not exclude tumor growth [11]. Visual loss is more common when post-chiasmal visual pathways are involved [12].

Nystagmus (vertical, horizontal, see-saw, rotary, dissociated pendular) may be the first sign of ONG/OCH, even before vision loss is noted. Spasmus nutans (pendular nystagmus, head nodding, and head tilt) may also be the first indication of ONG/OCH [13]. See Table 9-1 for a complete list of clinical signs and symptoms of ONG.

INVESTIGATIONS

Computed tomography (CT) and magnetic resonance imaging (MRI) have been used extensively in evaluating ONG/OCH (Figures 9-1 and 9-2). Long Tl and T2 relaxation times and intense contrast enhancement have been described [13,14]. However, these lesions may be isodense with surrounding tissues, even with T2 sequences or after gadolinium enhancement. Wilson [9] points out that ONGs sometimes appear to have a surrounding ring of increased signal on T2 sequences, especially when associated with NF-1. Cyst formation is rare [15], but is much more common in those without NF-1 [16]. The orbital optic nerve is more frequently involved in those patients with NF-1 than in those without NF-1 (66% vs. 32%) [16]. Coakley and coworkers [17] have proved pathologically that tumor limit as defined by MRI appearance does not correlate well with microscopic invasion, which was noted to be more extensive in 64% of their cases.

TREATMENT

The extensive literature up to 1994 is summarized by Dutton [1]. In general, definitive surgery is reserved for unilateral ONG with blindness or severe proptosis, or when the tumor appears to be extending to the chiasm. A group of patients with pilocytic astrocytomas treated with "conservative" surgery or no surgery combined with irradiation and chemotherapy had a 10-year survival rate of 85% [18]. A major issue is the well-documented observation that optic pathway gliomas may spontaneously resolve whether or not they are associated with NF-1 [19,20].

The literature on radiation therapy is extremely diverse, and the use of this modality needs to be individualized. It is usually reserved for those with chiasmal involvement and progression. Severe complications of radiation therapy in children, including intellectual impairment and growth hormone deficiency, are well recognized [2]. For example, Warman and colleagues [21] reported the case of a 10-year-old girl with a biopsy-proven pilocytic astrocytoma involving the OCH — visual

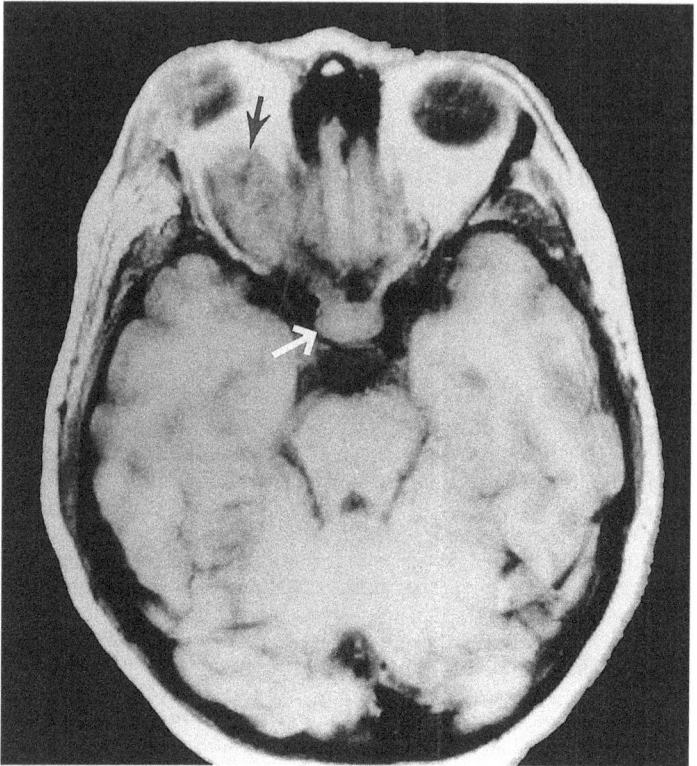

Fig. 9-1 Optic nerve with chiasmal glioma in T1-weighted unenhanced magnetic resonance imaging. *Black arrow* indicates intraorbital portion. *White arrow* shows thickened optic chiasm.

function was normal at presentation. Eight months after receiving 5,400 cGy of radiation therapy, she went totally blind from radiation necrosis of the visual pathways. Fractionated stereotactic radiation therapy seems to lessen complications [22].

Malignant transformation of benign tumors has also been reported after irradiation [1,7,8] (see Case Study), and radiation-induced neovascularization has been described [2,23].

Chemotherapy for progressive ONG/OCH is becoming more common for selected cases and may delay the use of radiation therapy with its attendant complications in children [24-31].

CASE STUDY

A 25-year-old man was seen in January 1988, complaining of fluctuating vision loss in his only functioning eye for 10 days. Patient history revealed that, when the patient was 4 years old, Frank B. Walsh, M.D., at the Wilmer Eye Institute,

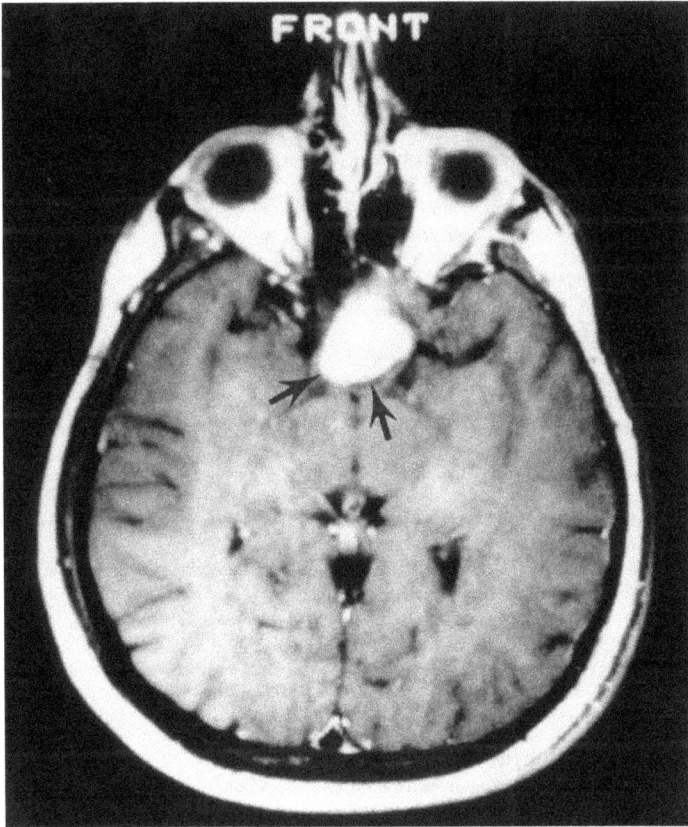

Fig. 9-2 Malignant transformation of formerly benign chiasmal glioma (*black arrows*) in T1-weighted gadolinium-enhanced magnetic resonance imaging. (See Case Study for clinical details.)

diagnosed a left ONG/OCH. The tumor was resected from the back of the globe to the optic chiasm, leaving the patient with a relative upper temporal field defect in his right eye (junction scotoma of Traquair). The histologic diagnosis was low-grade "optic glioma." He was treated with 3,500 cGy and thereafter lived in perfect health until his visit in 1988. There was no history of neurofibromatosis. A CT scan in 1983 showed no evidence of tumor in the parasellar region.

At the 1988 examination, visual acuity was 20/20 OD and no light perception in his left eye. A complete temporal hemianopia was present in the right eye. He was treated with steroids with transient recovery of the inferior temporal visual field. CT and MRI (see Figure 9-2) showed an enhancing suprasellar tumor, which proved to be an anaplastic astrocytoma.

Despite neurosurgery, radiation therapy, and brachytherapy, he went completely blind and died within 1 year.

Comment

This is an unfortunate example of malignant transformation of a formerly benign optochiasmatic glioma. In light of recent reports, the role of previous radiation therapy is suspect in this case [5,6].

REFERENCES

1. Dutton JJ. Gliomas of the anterior visual pathways. Surv Ophthalmol 1994;38:427.
2. Mapstone TB. Brain tumors in children. In Tomsak RL (ed), Pediatric Neuro-Ophthalmology. Boston: Butterworth-Heinemann, 1995;77.
3. Parazzini C, Triulzi E, Agnetti BV, et al. Spontaneous involution of optic pathway lesions in neurofibromatosis type 1: serial contrast MR evaluation. AJNR 1995;16:1711.
4. Singhal S, Birch JM, Kerr B, et al. Neurofibromatosis type 1 and sporadic optic glioma. Arch Dis Child 2002;87:65.
5. Grill J, Laithier V, Rodriguez D, et al. When do children with optic pathway tumors need treatment? An oncological perspective in 106 patients treated in a single center. Eur J Pediatr 2000;159:692.
6. Bruggers CS, Friedman HS, Phillips PC, et al. Leptomeningeal dissemination of optic pathway gliomas in three children. Am J Ophthalmol 1991;111:719.
7. Dirks PB, Jay V, Becker LE, et al. Development of anaplastic changes in low-grade astrocytomas of childhood. Neurosurgery 1994;34:68.
8. Safneck JR, Napier LB, Halliday WC. Malignant astrocytoma of the optic nerve in a child. Can J Neurol Sci 1992;19:498.
9. Wilson WB. Optic nerve gliomas: treatment differences for the benign and malignant varieties. In Tusa RJ, Newman SA (eds), Neuro-Ophthalmological Disorders: Diagnostic Work-up and Management. New York: Marcel Dekker, 1995;163.
10. Brzowski AE, Bazan C, Mumma JV, et al. Spontaneous regression of optic glioma in a patient with neurofibromatosis. Neurology 1992;42:679.
11. Kuenzle C, Weissert M, Roulet E, et al. Follow-up of optic pathway gliomas in children with neurofibromatosis type 1. Neuropediatrics 1994;25:295.
12. Balcer LJ, Liu GT, Heller G, et al. Visual loss in children with neurofibromatosis type 1 and optic pathway gliomas: relation to tumor location and magnetic resonance imaging. Am J Ophthalmol 2001;131:442.
13. Tomsak RL, Dell'Osso LF. Eye movement disturbances in children. In Tomsak RL (ed), Pediatric Neuro-Ophthalmology. Boston: Butterworth-Heinemann, 1995;29.
14. Kollias SS, Barkovich AJ, Edwards MS. Magnetic resonance analysis of suprasellar tumors of childhood. Pediatr Neurosurg 1991;17:284.
15. Tekkok IH, Tahta K, Saglam S. Optic nerve glioma presenting as a huge intrasellar mass. J Neurosurg Sci 1994;38:137.
16. Kornreich L, Blaser S, Schwarz M, et al. Optic pathway glioma: correlation of imaging findings with the presence of neurofibromatosis. AJNR 2001;22:1963.
17. Coakley KJ, Huston J III, Scheithauer BW, et al. Pilocytic astrocytomas: well-demarcated magnetic resonance appearance despite frequent infiltration histologically. Mayo Clin Proc 1995;70:747.
18. Sutton LN, Molloy PT, Sernyak H, et al. Long-term outcome of hypothalamic/chiasmatic astrocytomas in children treated with conservative surgery. J Neurosurg 1995;83:583.
19. Parsa CF, Hoyt CS, Lesser RL, et al. Spontaneous regression of optic gliomas: thirteen cases documented by serial neuro-imaging. Arch Ophthalmol 2001;119:516.
20. Schmandt SM, Packer RJ, Vezina LG, Jane J. Spontaneous regression of low-grade astrocytomas in childhood. Pediatr Neurosurg 2000;32:132.

21. Warman R, Glaser JS, Quencer RM. Radionecrosis of optico-hypothalamic glioma. Neuroophthalmology 1989;9:219.

22. Debus J, Kocagoncu KO, Hoss A, et al. Fractionated stereotactic radiotherapy (FRST) for optic glioma. Int J Radiat Oncol Biol Phys 1999;44:243.

23. Epstein MA, Packer RJ, Rorke LB, et al. Vascular malformation with radiation vasculopathy after treatment of chiasmatic/hypothalamic glioma. Cancer 1992;70:887.

24. Chamberlain MC. Recurrent chiasmatic-hypothalamic glioma treated with oral etoposide. Arch Neurol 1995;52:509.

25. Janss AJ, Grundy R, Canaan A, et al. Optic pathway and hypothalamic/chiasmatic gliomas in children younger than age 5 years with a 6 year follow-up. Cancer 1995;75:1051.

26. Charrow J, Listernick R, Greenwald MJ, et al. Carboplatin-induced regression of an optic pathway tumor in a child with neurofibromatosis. Med Pediatr Oncol 1993;21:680.

27. Moghrabi A, Friedman HS, Burger PC, et al. Carboplatin treatment of progressive optic pathway gliomas to delay radiotherapy. J Neurosurg 1993;79:223.

28. Pons MA, Finlay JL, Walker RW, et al. Chemotherapy with vincristine (VCR) and etoposide (VP-16) in children with low-grade astrocytoma. J Neurooncol 1992;14:151.

29. Kretschmar CS, Linggood RM. Chemotherapeutic treatment of extensive optic pathway tumors in infants. J Neurooncol 1991;10:263.

30. Petronio J, Edwards MS, Prados M, et al. Management of chiasmal and hypothalamic gliomas of infancy and childhood with chemotherapy. J Neurosurg 1991;74:701.

31. Silva MM, Goldman S, Keating G, et al. Optic pathway hypothalamic gliomas in children under three years of age: the role of chemotherapy. Pediatr Neurosurg 2000;33:151.

10

Optic Nerve Sheath Meningiomas

OVERVIEW

Optic nerve sheath meningiomas (ONSMs) represent one-third of all primary optic nerve tumors according to Dutton [1]. The mean age at presentation is approximately 40 years, and women are affected more frequently than men for a ratio of approximately 2:1. ONSMs rarely occur in children. Although some think that ONSMs in young people are more aggressive [2,3], there appears to be little evidence for this opinion [1]. These tumors arise from arachnoid villi cap cells, are benign, and spread by local extension. The histologic pattern is either meningothelial or transitional, with the papillary type being extremely rare [4]. ONSMs grow between the dura and arachnoid and do not invade the optic nerve or orbital contents. They are almost always unilateral. The rare bilateral cases are either due to intracranial meningiomas with intracanalicular spread [5] or associated with neurofibromatosis type 2 [6]. The main differential diagnosis is optic glioma (see Chapter 9).

MAIN CLINICAL FEATURES

The classic presentation of ONSM is the triad of vision loss, optic atrophy, and opticociliary shunt vessels (Hoyt-Spenser vessels, retinochoroidal collaterals) on the surface of the optic disc (Figure 10-1). Vision loss is usually slow but most often relentlessly progressive. Transient vision obscurations occur in up to 14% of patients [1]. Pain is usually not a prominent finding, but may occur antecedent to loss of vision and suggests the misdiagnosis of inflammatory orbital pseudotumor [7]. Restriction of ocular motility is largely due to stiffening of the optic nerve sheath from tumor growth. The new vessels on the optic disc are shunts between the retinal and choroidal venous systems [8,9] and most likely occur because of chronic retinal venous obstruction from tumor compression. See Table 10-1 for a complete list of the signs and symptoms of ONSM.

INVESTIGATIONS

Computed tomography of the orbit is still an excellent tool for diagnosis of ONSM, with an accuracy rate of over 95% [1] (Figure 10-2). The "tram-track" sign — parallel tumor enhancement surrounding central optic nerve lucency — is present in approximately 20% of cases. A fusiform or globular shape is common. However, gadolinium-enhanced

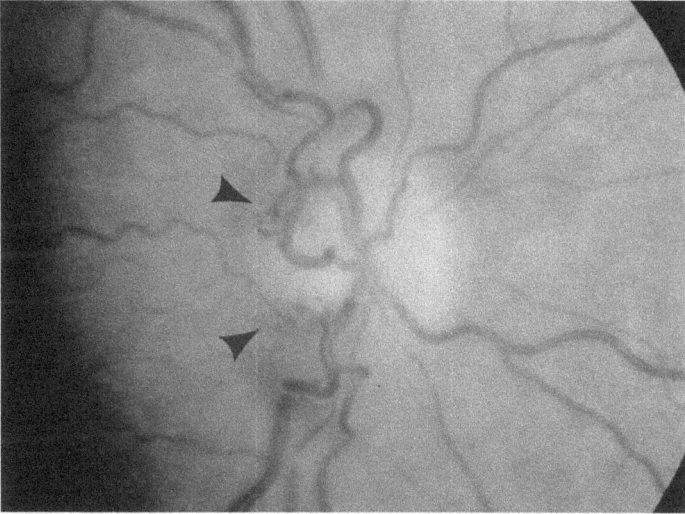

Fig. 10-1   Chronic disc edema with retinochoroidal collateral vessels (opticociliary shunts, Hoyt-Spencer vessels) *(arrowheads)* in patient with optic nerve sheath meningioma.

Table 10-1 Signs and Symptoms of Optic Nerve Sheath Meningiomas at Presentation	
Loss of visual acuity	96%
Visual field loss	83%
Dyschromatopsia	73%
Proptosis	59%
Optic atrophy	49%
Optic disc edema	48%
Opticociliary collateral vessels	30%
Decreased ocular motility	47%

Source: Dutton JJ. Optic nerve sheath meningiomas. Surv Ophthalmol 1992;37:167.

magnetic resonance imaging (MRI) — especially with fat suppression — is much more sensitive for detecting the extent of the tumor and the presence of intracranial growth [10,11]. Perioptic cyst formation behind the globe, as part of ONSM, has also been delineated with MRI [12].

Orbital echography demonstrates medium-to-high internal reflectivity and irregular acoustic structure of ONSM.

TREATMENT

Treatment for ONSM varies depending on the extent of tumor growth and degree of visual disability. Miller has recently emphasized that these tumors are not associated with mortality or significant neurologic dysfunction and rarely cause loss of vision in the fellow eye [13], and

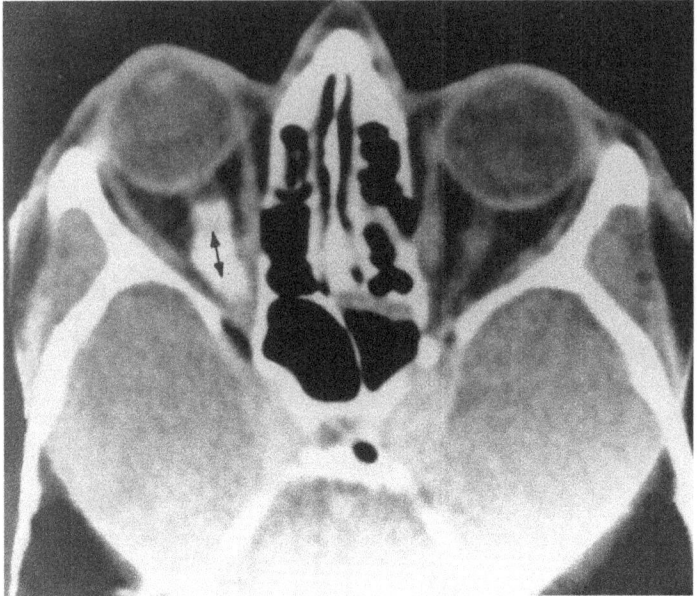

Fig. 10-2 Optic nerve sheath meningioma. Arrows indicate clacified area of tumor.

Dutton [1] points out that fatalities reported with ONSM are from surgical complications. However, in the past, surgical extirpation often was the treatment of choice if the tumor had caused blindness. In this setting orbitotomy with or without craniotomy is dictated by presence or absence of intracranial extension. Radiotherapy is often combined with surgery, especially when a subtotal resection of tumor is performed.

The older literature recommends more aggressive treatment in patients younger than 21 years of age [2,3], but more recent data do not confirm a worse prognosis in younger individuals with ONSM [1],

If useful vision remains, careful observation or conventional fractionated radiation therapy (approximately 5,500 cGy) are the most commonly recommended strategies [14-18]. In 1981, Smith and colleagues [18] described the palliative effect of radiation therapy on ONSM visual disability. Others have confirmed this finding, and now radiation therapy can be expected to improve or stabilize visual function for a minimum of 5 years in the majority of treated cases [1,14,16,17]. Complications from conventional radiation therapy of the optic nerve occur in approximately 16% of cases and include further visual field loss, central retinal artery occlusion, and encephalopathy [19].

Newer methods promise to improve results of radiation therapy. For example, Pitz and others treated 15 patients with stereotactic fractionated conformal irradiation and observed them for 3 years [20]. Visual field improved in six cases, visual acuity in one case, no visual deterioration was observed in any case, and significant complications were not found [20]. These findings led Miller to advocate this method as the preferred one for radiation therapy of ONSM [21].

Two other studies with smaller numbers or shorter follow-up times also showed promising results for stereotactic fractionated irradiation in the treatment of ONSM [22,23].

Hormone therapy and the measurement of steroid receptors have not been commonly used in the treatment of ONSM. However, a recent report found high levels of progesterone receptors in 30 ONSMs but not in benign meningiomas from other intracranial sites [24].

REFERENCES

1. Dutton JJ. Optic nerve sheath meningiomas. Surv Ophthalmol 1992;37:167.
2. Alper MG. Management of primary optic nerve meningiomas: current status-therapy in controversy. J Clin Neuroophthalmol 1981;1:101.
3. Wright JE, McNab AA, MacDonald WL. Primary optic nerve sheath meningiomas. Br J Ophthalmol 1989;73:960.
4. Shuangshoti S. Primary papillary meningioma of the optic nerve sheath: a case of unique location and benign pathology. Surg Neurol 1993;39:200.
5. Lewis T, Kingsley D, Mosely I. Do bilateral optic nerve sheath meningiomas exist? Br J Neurosurg 1991;5:13.
6. Cunliffe IA, Moffat DA, Hardy DG, et al. Bilateral optic nerve sheath meningioma in a patient with neurofibromatosis type 2. Br J Ophthalmol 1992;76:310.
7. Wroe SJ, Thompson AJ, McDonald WI. Painful intraorbital meningiomas. J Neurol Neurosurg Psychiatry 1991;54:1009.
8. Schatz H, Green WR, Talamo JH, et al. Clinicopathologic correlation of retinal to choroidal venous collaterals of the optic nerve head. Ophthalmology 1991;98:1287.
9. Muci-Mendoza R, Arevalo JF, Ramella M, et al. Optociliary veins in optic nerve sheath meningioma. Indocyanine green videoangiography findings. Ophthalmology 1999;106:311.
10. Zimmerman CF, Schatz NJ, Glaser JS. Magnetic resonance imaging of optic nerve meningioma. Ophthalmology 1990;97:585.
11. Lindblom B, Truwit CL, Hoyt WF. Optic nerve sheath meningioma. Definition of intraorbital, intracanalicular, and intracranial components with magnetic resonance imaging. Ophthalmology 1992;99:560.
12. Lindblom B, Norman D, Hoyt WF. Perioptic cyst distal to optic nerve meningioma: MR demonstration. AJNR Am J Neuroradiol 1992;13:1622.
13. Miller NR. Radiation for optic nerve meningiomas: Is this the answer? Ophthalmology 2002;109:833.
14. Kennerdell JS, Maroon JC, Malton M, et al. The management of optic nerve sheath meningiomas. Am J Ophthalmol 1988;106:450.
15. Burde RM, Smith JL. Editorial comment: spontaneous reduction of growth rate of a large intracranial meningioma. J Clin Neuroophthalmol 1984;4:137.
16. Maroon JC, Kennerdell JS, Vidovich DV, et al. Recurrent spheno-orbital meningioma. J Neurosurg 1994;80:202.
17. Turbin RE, Thompson CR, Kennerdell JS, et al. A long-term visual outcome comparison in patients with optic nerve sheath meningioma managed with observation, surgery, radiotherapy, or surgery and radiotherapy. Ophthalmology 2002;109:890.

18. Smith JL, Vuksanovic MM, Yates BM, et al. Radiation therapy for primary optic nerve meningiomas. J Clin Neuroophthalmol 1981;1:85.
19. Capo H, Kupersmith MJ. Efficacy and complications of radiotherapy of anterior visual pathway tumors. Neurol Clin 1991;9:179.
20. Pitz S, Becker G, Schiefer U, et al. Stereotactic fractionated irradiation of optic nerve sheath meningioma: a new treatment alternative. Br J Ophthalmol 2002;86:1265.
21. Miller NR. The evolving management of optic nerve sheath meningiomas. Br J Ophthalmol 2002;86:1198.
22. Liu JK, Forman S, Hershewe GL, et al. Optic nerve sheath meningiomas: visual improvement after stereotactic radiotherapy. Neurosurgery 2002;50:950.
23. Andrews DW, Faroozan R, Yang BP, et al. Fractionated stereotactic radiotherapy for the treatment of optic nerve sheath meningiomas: preliminary observations of 33 optic nerves in 30 patients with historical comparison to observation with or without prior surgery. Neurosurgery 2002;51:890.
24. Thom M, Martinian L. Progesterone receptors are expressed with higher frequency by optic nerve sheath meningiomas. Clin Neuropathol 2002;21:5.

11

Optic Neuritis

OVERVIEW AND ETIOLOGY

Optic neuritis is a common optic nerve disorder usually affecting individuals between the ages of 15 and 45. Women are affected approximately three times more frequently than men. The pathogenesis is related to inflammation and demyelination, regardless of whether multiple sclerosis (MS) is present. Optic neuritis may be classified anatomically (e.g., retrobulbar optic neuritis, papillitis, neuroretinitis) or by incidence (retrobulbar being the most common, followed by papillitis and neuroretinitis), or related to etiology (MS, followed by idiopathic/post-viral, collagen vascular, syphilis, sarcoid, etc.) [1]. The results of the Optic Neuritis Treatment Trial (ONTT) have shed new light on the clinical profile, natural history, and treatment of the disease, and these results are the focus of this discussion.

USUAL CLINICAL FEATURES

Kestenbaum [2] stated that "the lesion of the central vision is usually the first, the most severe, and the last sign of the disease."

The relative afferent pupillary defect (RAPD, Marcus Gunn pupil), which documents a difference in conduction between optic nerves, may not be present if the optic neuritis is bilateral.

The ONTT analyzed visual field measurements made on the Humphrey automated perimeter (Allergan, Irvine, CA) (central 30 degrees) and found diffuse abnormalities in the central visual field in about 48% of affected eyes. Localized defects were altitudinal in 15% and quadrantic in 13%, followed by lower numbers of miscellaneous defects. Chiasmal defects were present in 5% and retrochiasmal defects were noted in 9% [3]. Approximately two thirds of asymptomatic fellow eyes had slight visual field abnormalities at presentation.

Box 11-1   Usual Clinical Features of Optic Neuritis

Unilateral loss of central vision over hours to days
Relative afferent pupillary defect
Diffuse or localized visual field defects affecting the central visual field
Dyschromatopsia
Pain on eye movement
Other: diminished contrast sensitivity (98%); photopsias (30%)
Excellent prognosis for visual recovery over months

Color vision abnormalities, as tested with Ishihara color plates or the FM-100 hue test, were present in 88-94% [4].

Pain on eye movement was present in 92% (mild, 51%; moderate, 36%; severe, 13%). Despite the high prevalence of pain, it is infrequently a volunteered complaint.

See Box 11-1 for a complete list of the usual clinical features of optic neuritis.

NATURAL HISTORY OF VISUAL DYSFUNCTION
Ninety-five percent of untreated patients in the ONTT had a visual acuity of 20/40 or better after 1 year of follow-up [5]. Visual improvement usually began within the first month after onset of symptoms. Severity of initial vision loss (i.e., 20/200 or worse) was somewhat predictive of a poorer vision prognosis [6].

Visual field also improves significantly over time and improvement does not seem to be dependent on the initial type of field loss [7]. Five-year follow-up analysis of visual function showed that 87% of patients had visual acuities of 20/25 or better. Recurrent optic neuritis (same or fellow eye) occurred in 28% of patients during the 5-year period but prognosis for visual improvement was excellent in this group as well. Recurrent optic neuritis was more common in patients with clinically definite MS (CDMS) and in those who had received only oral prednisone treatment [8].

DIFFERENTIAL DIAGNOSIS
Conditions that may mimic retrobulbar optic neuritis include compressive optic neuropathies, autoimmune optic neuropathies, radiation-induced optic neuropathy, paraneoplastic optic neuropathies, and central serous choroidopathy.

Optic nerve diseases that may be confused with papillitis include Leber's hereditary optic neuropathy, diabetic papillopathy, venous stasis retinopathy, impending central retinal vein occlusion, ischemic optic neuropathy, and optic nerve drusen [9].

INVESTIGATIONS
A complete neuro-ophthalmologic examination, emphasizing visual acuity at near and far distances, a search for the RAPD, color vision testing, and careful perimetry are essential in evaluating optic neuritis. Initial analysis of ONTT data led to the conclusion that the use of ancillary studies (antinuclear antibodies, fluorescent treponemal antibody absorption test, chest x-ray, lumbar puncture, and magnetic resonance imaging [MRI]) was limited for defining a cause for vision loss other than optic neuritis associated with demyelinating disease [4]. The overall incidence of white matter lesions found with MRI was 48.7%.

However, subgroup analysis showed that 36% of placebo group patients with two or more periventricular lesions, of at least 3 mm in size identified by MRI, developed CDMS within 2 years, compared with only 3% of those in whom MRI was normal.

A more recent longitudinal study of abnormalities on MRI and disability from MS spanned more than 14 years [10]. These patients were entered because of isolated symptoms clinically suggestive of MS (e.g., optic neuritis, brainstem and spinal cord involvement). After 14.1 years 88% of patients with MRI involvement on initial scan had CDMS whereas only 19% of those with a normal initial scan had developed CDMS. Therefore, the results of the ONTT and other studies are consistent in showing that MRI is the most important test regarding the risk of developing CDMS after optic neuritis or other monosymptomatic neurological events consistent with demyelination.

The predictive value of cerebrospinal fluid oligoclonal banding for the development of CDMS was recently found to be of use only in those patients who had no MRI lesions at the time of presentation of optic neuritis [11].

TREATMENT

In the ONTT, 457 patients with optic neuritis were randomized to receive either (1) placebo, (2) oral prednisone (OP) (1 mg/kg/day for 14 days), or (3) intravenous methylprednisolone (IVMP) (250 mg every 6 hours for 12 doses) followed by OP (1 mg/kg/day for 11 days). Visual acuity at 1 year was 20/40 or better in 95% of the placebo group, 94% in the IVMP group, and 91% in the OP group. Surprisingly, recurrent attacks of optic neuritis or new attacks in the fellow eye were highest in the OP group (relative risk: 1.83 for the OP group vs. 0.95 for the IVMP group). This finding has led to the recommendation that OP not be used in the treatment of optic neuritis. However, this conclusion only holds for the specific dose and duration of treatment used in the study.

As noted in the section on Investigations, patients with white matter lesions detected with MRI have a greater chance of developing CDMS within 2 years. The ONTT showed that treatment of this subgroup of patients with a combination of IVMP and OP reduced the 2-year incidence of CDMS by more than 50% [12]. However, 5-year follow-up data showed an overall cumulative probability of developing CDMS of 30%, and this risk did not differ by treatment group [13]. Results of MRI was a strong predictor of CDMS with the 5-year risk being approximately 16% in patients with no MRI lesions to 51% in those with three or more MRI lesions at the time of presentation. Taken together, these findings suggest that the protective effect of one ONTT treatment cycle wanes after approximately 2 years. Could repeated pulses of IV methylprednisone be effective in retarding signs and symptoms of MS? This possibility was investigated by Zivadinov and colleagues in patients with relapsing-remitting MS [14]. They found that scheduled pulses of IV methylprednisolone three times a year for 3 years followed by twice a year for 2 years slowed development of MRI T1 "black holes," whole brain atrophy, and disability score worsening when compared to control patients pulsed only at the time of relapses.

Other drugs appear to be useful in preventing the progression of MS. The Controlled High-Risk Subjects Avonex Multiple Sclerosis Prevention Study (CHAMPS) compared weekly interferon beta-1a injections to placebo injections in patients at high risk for development of CDMS over 3 years. Both groups were treated once initially with the ONTT IV-oral steroid protocol. Serial MRIs were done every 6 months as were clinical examinations. The rates of developing CDMS in patients presenting with optic neuritis (28% vs. 37%), as well as a salutary effect on MRI parameters, were better in the interferon group at a level of statistical significance [15].

Based on this new evidence, my (RT) recommendation for evaluation and treatment of optic neuritis is as follows: (1) perform MRI for all new patients with isolated optic neuritis; and (2) suggest treatment with a combination of IVMP and OP in the following circumstances: (a) if MRI is suggestive of MS, regardless of visual acuity, or (b) if presenting visual acuity is 20/200 or worse, or if speedy resolution of visual dysfunction is a prime concern, even if MRI is normal; (3) offer combination IV oral steroid treatment to those with optic neuritis and a negative MRI; (4) refer patient to a neurologist who is facile with the treatment of MS for a baseline exam and consideration of treatment with immunomodulating drugs.

REFERENCES

1. Miller NR. Demyelinating diseases: optic neuritis. In Tusa RJ, Newman SA (eds), Neuro-Ophthalmological Disorders: Diagnostic Work-up and Management. New York: Marcel Dekker, 1995;27.
2. Kestenbaum A. Clinical Methods of Neuro-Ophthalmologic Examination (2nd ed). New York: Grune & Stratton, 1961;135.
3. Keltner JL, Johnson CA, Spurr JO, et al. Visual field profile of optic neuritis: one-year follow-up in the optic neuritis treatment trial. Arch Ophthalmol 1994;112:946.
4. Optic Neuritis Study Group. The clinical profile of optic neuritis. Arch Ophthalmol 1991;109:1673.
5. Beck RW, Cleary PA. Optic neuritis treatment trial: one-year follow-up results. Arch Ophthalmol 1993;111:773.
6. Beck RW, Cleary PA, Backlund JC. The course of visual recovery after optic neuritis: experience of the optic neuritis treatment trial. Ophthalmology 1994;101:1771.
7. Fang JP, Lin RH, Donohue SP. Recovery of visual field function in the optic neuritis treatment trial. Am J Ophthalmol 1999;128:566.
8. Optic Neuritis Study Group. Visual function 5 years after optic neuritis: experience of the Optic Neuritis Treatment Trial. Arch Ophthalmol 1997;115:1545.
9. Sedwick LA. Optic neuritis. Neurol Clin 1991;9:97.
10. Brex PA, Ciccarelli O, O'Riordan JI, et al. A longitudinal study of abnormalities on MRI and disability from multiple sclerosis. N Engl J Med 2002;346:158.
11. Cole SR, Beck RW, Moke PS, et al. The predictive value of CSF oligoclonal banding for MS 5 years after optic neuritis. Neurology 1998;51:885.
12. Trobe JD. High-dose corticosteroid regimen retards development of multiple sclerosis in optic neuritis treatment trial [editorial]. Arch Ophthalmol 1994;112:35.
13. Optic Neuritis Study Group. The 5-year risk of MS after optic neuritis. Experience of the optic neuritis treatment trial. Neurology 1997;49:1404.
14. Zivadinov R, Rudick RA, De Masi R, et al. Effects of IV methylprednisolone on brain atrophy in relapsing-remitting MS. Neurology 2001;57:1239.
15. CHAMPS Study Group. Interferon beta-1a for optic neuritis patients at high risk for multiple sclerosis. Am J Ophthalmol 2001;132:463.

12

Pseudotumor Cerebri (Idiopathic Intracranial Hypertension)

OVERVIEW AND ETIOLOGY

Pseudotumor cerebri (PTC; also commonly called idiopathic intracranial hypertension; IIH) is an enigmatic disorder of increased cerebrospinal fluid (CSF) pressure whose major symptoms, signs, and complications affect the visual system. The pathogenesis of this condition is somewhat controversial and probably multifactorial. However, impaired CSF absorption through abnormal arachnoid granulations or cerebral venous hypertension are the most likely major factors for elevation of intracranial pressure (ICP) [1-4]. In approximately 50% of cases, PTC occurs in isolation, although numerous conditions and exogenous agents have been associated with its development, especially obesity, rapid weight gain, vitamin A ingestion [5], oral tetracycline use [6,7], sleep apnea [8], and partial [9] or complete cerebral venous sinus thrombosis or collapse [10]. Pediatric PTC is less often associated with obesity than is PTC in adults [11,12]. Obesity has been hypothesized to elevate cerebral venous pressure by increasing intra-abdominal pressure and thereby impeding venous return from the brain to the heart [13,14]. Women are affected 2-5 times more frequently with PTC than men, but men seem to have visual complications more often and with more severity [15].

MAIN CLINICAL FEATURES

The major clinical symptoms and signs of PTC are listed in Tables 12-1 and 12-2 and Box 12-1.

The headache associated with PTC is often similar to episodic tension type headache or to migraine without aura [16], although orthostatic

Table 12-1 Major Clinical Symptoms of Pseudotumor Cerebri	
Headache	91%
Vision loss	39%
Transient vision obscurations	36%
Horizontal diplopia	34%
Pulsatile intracranial noises	28%
Pain with eye movement	22%

Sources: Giuseffi V, Wall M, Siegel PZ, et al. Symptoms and disease associations in idiopathic intracranial hypertension (pseudotumor cerebri): a case-control study. Neurology 1991;41:239; and Smith JL. Pseudotumor cerebri. Trans Am Acad Ophthalmol Otolaryngol 1958;62:432.

Table 12-2 Minor Clinical Symptoms of Pseudotumor Cerebri	
Neck stiffness	31%
Paresthesias	22%
Arthralgias	13%
Back and leg pain	5%
Ataxia	4%

Source: Round R, Keane JR. The minor symptoms of increased intracranial pressure: 101 patients with benign intracranial hypertension. Neurology 1988;38:1461.

components are quite common. There is evidence that ICP elevation per se is not the cause for the pain [17]. Transient visual obscurations are episodes of vision loss that last seconds and most likely occur from a combination of optic nerve ischemia secondary to papilledema and stasis of axoplasmic transport [18]. In the majority of cases, permanent vision loss results from optic atrophy secondary to chronic papilledema. Isolated cases of vision loss in PTC have been attributed to subretinal hemorrhage from peripapillary subretinal choroidal neovascular membranes, to anterior ischemic optic neuropathy, or to macular changes [19,20]. In some patients with PTC, acquired hyperopia with choroidal folds develops in response to flattening of the posterior aspect of the globe [21]. Pulsatile intracranial noises are abolished by jugular compression.

Papilledema results from elevated ICP being transmitted to the retrolaminar portion of the optic nerve via the subarachnoid space. The absence of papilledema [22,23] or the presence of asymmetric or unilateral papilledema in PTC is best explained by anatomic variants in the optic nerve subarachnoid space effectively walling off the retrolaminar region of the optic nerve from elevated ICP [18].

Vision loss takes many forms. Loss of Snellen acuity tends to be mild in the majority of series reported. For example, Wall and George [24] found that only 13% of 50 patients with PTC had acuities less than 20/20 on initial examination. This had decreased to 10% by the final visit. Loss of contrast sensitivity occurs in 50-75% of patients with PTC and is a sensitive parameter correlating well with permanent vision loss [24]. Visual field loss takes many forms (Table 12-3). Early changes occur within the central 30 degrees of visual field [25].

It is apparent from the foregoing that many patients with PTC have visual field loss without loss of visual acuity. In those reports that address loss of visual function in toto, more than half of all patients with

Box 12-1   Main Clinical Findings of Pseudotumor Cerebri
Papilledema
Loss of visual function
Visual acuity
Color vision
Contrast sensitivity
Visual field
Ocular motility disturbances
Unilateral or bilateral sixth cranial nerve palsies

Table 12-3 Visual Field Loss in Pseudotumor Cerebri	
Enlargement of blind spot	≥90%
Concentric constriction	40%
Inferonasal depressions	18%
Arcuate defects	10%
Cecocentral scotomas	10%

Source: Tomsak RL, Sweeney PJ. Pseudotumor cerebri: some neuro-ophthalmologic perspectives. In Daroff RB, Conomy JP (eds), Contributions to Contemporary Neurology: A Tribute to Joseph M. Foley. Stoneham, MA: Butterworth, 1988;201.

PTC sustain some permanent loss of sight [24,26,27]. Ocular motility disturbances are most often unilateral or bilateral sixth cranial nerve palsies of mild degree. These are thought to be a nonlocalizing finding caused by increased ICP. Other cranial nerve dysfunction (third, fourth, seventh) has been reported with PTC, but these cases are so rare that other causes of cranial neuropathy should first be excluded [2,28-30].

OFFICE EVALUATION OF PSEUDOTUMOR CEREBRI

The important points in the clinical examination of a patient with PTC are summarized in Box 12-2.

INVESTIGATIONS

Investigations for PTC are based on the modified Dandy criteria for diagnosis (Box 12-3). An update of this schema has been published recently [31]. Note that neuroimaging and CSF evaluation are required to exclude other causes for increased ICP. Computed tomography or magnetic resonance imaging (MRI) is used to rule out mass lesions. A number of MRI findings have been reported in PTC, including flattening of the posterior sclera (80% prevalence), empty sella (70% prevalence), distention of the optic nerve sheaths (45% prevalence), contrast enhancement of the prelaminar optic nerve (50% prevalence), vertical

Box 12-2   Office Evaluation of Pseudotumor Cerebri
Patient history
Headache
Vision loss, transient visual obscurations, diplopia
Rapid weight gain
Endocrine problems (e.g., menstrual irregularities)
Medications, vitamins (e.g., vitamin A, tetracycline)
Visual acuity (best corrected, distance and near)
Color vision
Contrast sensitivity
Amsler grid examination
Perimetry (automated and/or kinetic)
Pupillary evaluation
Funduscopy (after mydriasis)
Fundus photography

> **Box 12-3   Modified Dandy Criteria for Diagnosis of Pseudotumor Cerebri**
>
> Signs and symptoms of increased intracranial pressure
> Absence of finding on neurologic examination except for papilledema and occasional sixth cranial nerve palsies
> No sign of mass or enlarged ventricles on neuroimaging
> Normal cerebrospinal fluid composition

Sources: Dandy WE. Intracranial pressure without brain tumour: diagnosis and treatment. Ann Surg 1937;106;492 and Smith JL. Whence pseudotumor cerebri? J Clin Neuro-ophthalmol 1985;5:55.

tortuosity of the intraorbital optic nerve (40% prevalence), and elevation of the prelaminar optic nerve (30% prevalence) [32]. Cerebral venous sinus thrombosis can be diagnosed by MRI if special attention is paid to the venous circulation [33], but the prevalence of venous sinus thrombosis in uncomplicated PTC is low [34]. Visual-evoked potentials are of limited use in diagnosing or following patients with PTC [35].

TREATMENT FOR PSEUDOTUMOR CEREBRI

The primary goal in PTC treatment is to preserve or restore visual function by permanently lowering ICP or by protecting the retrolaminar portion of the eye from elevated ICP.

Pharmacologic Therapy for Pseudotumor Cerebri

Inhibition of CSF production is the goal of most medical therapy for PTC, because no drugs are available that enhance CSF outflow. Of the carbonic anhydrase inhibitors, acetazolamide (Diamox) is the drug of choice. A dose of 20 mg/kg maximally inhibits CSF production in rats. For a 70-kg person this would equal 1,400 mg/day; obviously, the dose would be higher in an obese person if this relationship holds for humans. Side effects include anorexia, malaise, paresthesias, and altered taste, especially for carbonated beverages. Acetazolamide can also cause hypokalemia and kidney stones. Side effects can be minimized by using the slow-release form of acetazolamide (Diamox Sequels) [36]. Acetazolamide has proved effective in some patients with PTC [37]. Other carbonic anhydrase inhibitors (e.g., methazolamide [Neptazane]) are often used in acetazolamide-intolerant patients, but their efficacy has not been proved.

Furosemide (Lasix) also inhibits CSF production and may have an additive effect with acetazolamide, at least in experimental animals [38]. This drug has not been systematically studied in PTC, but it is used by experts in the field [18].

Topiramate, an antiepileptic agent with anorectic effects, also is a weak carbonic anhydrase inhibitor. It has been used successfully at a dose of 100 mg/day in divided doses to treat PTC [39].

Corticosteroids are not a first-line treatment for PTC but may be used in selective cases. Fishman [38] notes that these drugs do not alter CSF dynamics but rather decrease brain edema by other mechanisms. Short-term high-dose intravenous (IV) or oral steroids may be a useful adjunctive therapy (see Case Study). Liu and coworkers [40] treated patients with severe papilledema and acute vision loss from PTC with IV methylprednisolone and acetazolamide with good results. Again, the use of steroids, carbonic anhydrase inhibitors, and/or diuretics mandates timely measurement of serum electrolytes.

Digoxin, in standard cardiac doses, has been used successfully to treat PTC in a small group of patients [41].

Indomethacin lowers CSF pressure, cerebral blood flow, and cerebrovascular permeability, although it is not commonly used for the treatment of PTC [17].

The subject of medical treatment of PTC should not be concluded without a discussion of weight reduction. Newborg [42] studied nine patients with PTC placed on a salt-restricted, rapid weight-reduction rice diet. All showed improvement in papilledema. Their mean weight was 261 pounds before treatment and 187 pounds after treatment. This worked out to an average monthly weight loss of 15 pounds. Indeed, one subject lost 65 pounds in 2 months and another lost 60 pounds in 3 months! My (RT) interpretation of these results is that rapidity of the weight loss, rather than the return to "normal" weight, beneficially influenced PTC in these patients. More recently Johnson and co-workers found that loss of 6% of body weight over a 24-week period had a salutary effect on papilledema from PTC when combined with acetazolamide therapy [43].

Surgical Treatment for Pseudotumor Cerebri

In Dandy's era, subtemporal decompression was the treatment of choice for elevated ICP and brain swelling [44]. Today, optic nerve sheath decompression (ONSD) and lumbar-peritoneal shunts are popular.

Historically, repeated lumbar punctures were advocated for the treatment of PTC, especially in children, although the reasons for this procedure's effectiveness are unclear in light of CSF dynamics. Fishman [38] points out that CSF formation occurs at a rate of approximately 500 ml per day, which means that the CSF compartment would be reconstituted within hours, even if completely drained. It is possible that repeated taps at the same lumbar level create a fistula with drainage into the epidural space. Corbett [28] cautions about the complication of intraspinal epidermoid tumors resulting from repeated lumbar punctures. This treatment is almost never used today except occasionally in managing PTC during pregnancy.

Lumbar-peritoneal shunting has the benefit of reducing ICP, thus treating papilledema, diplopia, and headaches. Complications such as shunt migration, infection, shunt breakage, and malposition occur in approximately 10% of cases [45]. Shunt failure (55%) and low-pressure headaches (21%) occurred frequently in one series [46]. Others have had a more positive experience with this procedure [47,48].

Optic nerve sheath decompression is the treatment of choice of most neuro-ophthalmologists. Some variation of the following procedure is used by most surgeons: (1) a transconjunctival medial orbitotomy is performed; (2) the medial rectus muscle is isolated and removed from the globe; (3) after abducting the eye and careful retraction, the optic nerve is identified under the operating microscope and its dura is incised and excised to form a window through which CSF egresses into the orbit; and (4) medial rectus muscle and conjunctiva are reposited at their normal locations. Lateral orbital approaches to the optic nerve are favored by some [49,50]. The use of the antimetabolite mitomycin and a Molteno valve has also been reported as a modification of ONSD [51].

ONSD leads to resolution of papilledema and visual improvement on the ipsilateral side in 70-97% of cases [52-55]. The mechanism for its long-term salutary effect is not permanent diversion of CSF into the orbit, but rather the formation of circumferential adhesions between the dura and the optic nerve, which wall off the laminar region from the CSF pressure head [56-59] and potentially improve optic disc blood flow [49,60]. It may also be that fenestration of the nerve sheath alters the fluid dynamics such that pressure at the laminar level is diminished [61]. If needed, ONSD can be used in patients with lumbar-peritoneal shunts and persistent papilledema [62]. Complications are rare but may be severe. For example, in one series of 200 patients, three lost vision from retinal or optic nerve complications of ONSD [63]. Transient vision loss has also been described following ONSD [64]. Less severe complications, such as diplopia, corneal dellen, and dacryocystitis, occurred approximately 12% of the time in this series [63].

Gastric surgery to induce weight loss in obese patients with PTC has also led to a resolution of signs and symptoms [13,14].

Venous sinus stenting was used successfully in one woman with PTC who had partial obstruction of both transverse sinuses [65].

CASE STUDY

A 27-year-old obese woman was referred for management of PTC. She complained of daily headaches of moderate severity. Her visual acuity on initial examination was 20/20 OU. The neuro-ophthalmologic examination was normal except for papilledema bilaterally and slightly depressed visual fields (Octopus 123 G1X program [Interzeag, Switzerland]; mean sensitivities: 24.5 dB OD and 25.8 dB OS). She was treated initially with acetazolamide (Diamox), 500 mg twice per day, but could not tolerate the side effects. She was switched to methazolamide (Neptazane), 50 mg three times per day, and the headaches were treated with propranolol (Inderal), 80 mg twice per day, and nortriptyline (Pamelor), 50 mg at bedtime. The papilledema resolved and visual fields improved gradually in the right eye so that, 2 years later, the mean sensitivities were 28.3 dB OD and 25.8 dB OS.

However, a few months later, she was seen with complaints of "dark circles" in her vision. She denied any change in her health, weight, or medications. Visual acuity was 20/25 OU at far distances and JI at near. She missed the temporal number of the double-digit Ishihara color plates with the right eye and missed eight plates with the left eye. Papilledema had returned (Figure 12-1). Visual fields showed a temporal paracentral scotoma in the right eye with a mean sensitivity of 24.4 dB and a dense inferonasal defect in the left eye (mean sensitivity: 20.4 dB) (Figure 12-2). She was treated with prednisone, 100 mg per day, for 10 days and

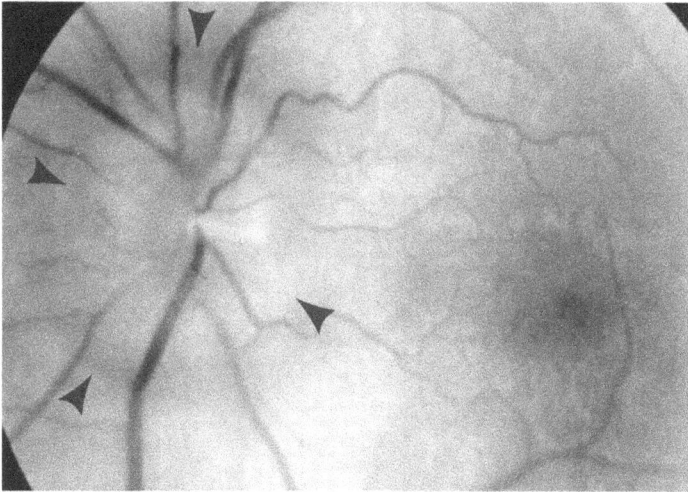

Fig. 12-1 Recurrent papilledema in the left eye of a patient with pseudotumor cerebri. Arrowheads outline extent of disc edema.

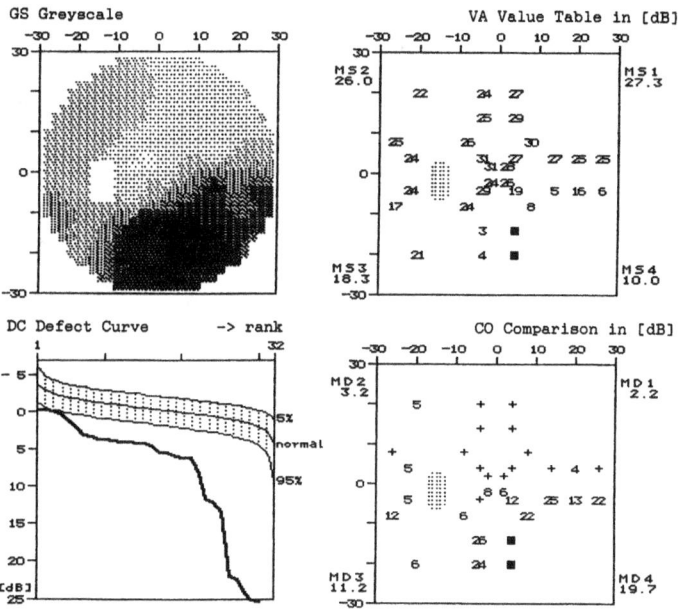

Fig. 12-2 Visual field corresponding to Figure 12-1 Octopus 123 modified G1X program (Interzeag, Switzerland). Mean sensitivity is 20.4 dB.

GS Greyscale

-30 -20 -10 0 10 20 30

VA Value Table in [dB]

-30 -20 -10 0 10 20 30

MS2 28.9   MS1 29.4

25   28 29
            29 29
29   28   30
30   31 31   29 29 27
        32 32
23   29 29   23 22 19
23   28   26
        17 13
MS3 24.9   27   20 14   MS4 22.3

DC Defect Curve   -> rank

1   32

-5
0
5
10
15
20
[dB]
25

5%
normal
95%

CO Comparison in [dB]

-30 -20 -10 0 10 20 30

MD2 0.2   MD1 0.0

+   + +
        + +
    +   +
+   + +   + + +
6   + +   7 7 9
6   +
    12 15
MD3 4.4   +   8 14   MD4 7.3

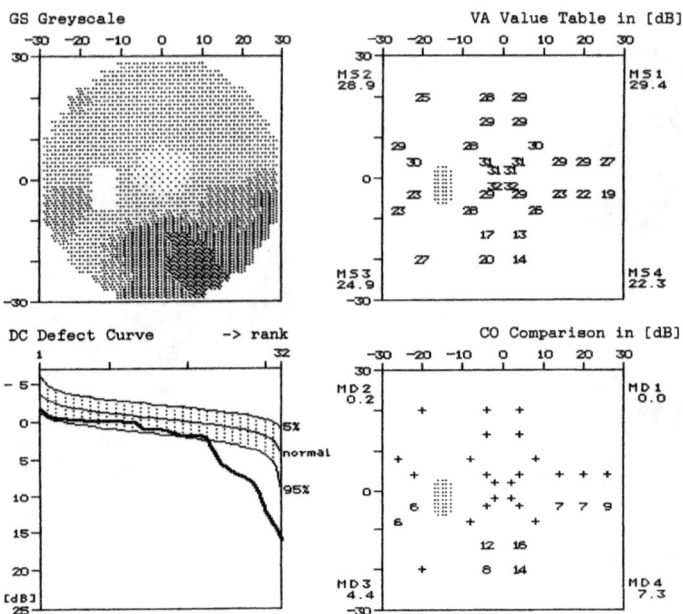

Fig. 12-3 Visual field corresponding to Figure 12-4 and showing partial resolution of field detect. Octopus 123 modified G1X program (Interzeag, Switzerland). Mean sensitivity is 26.3 dB.

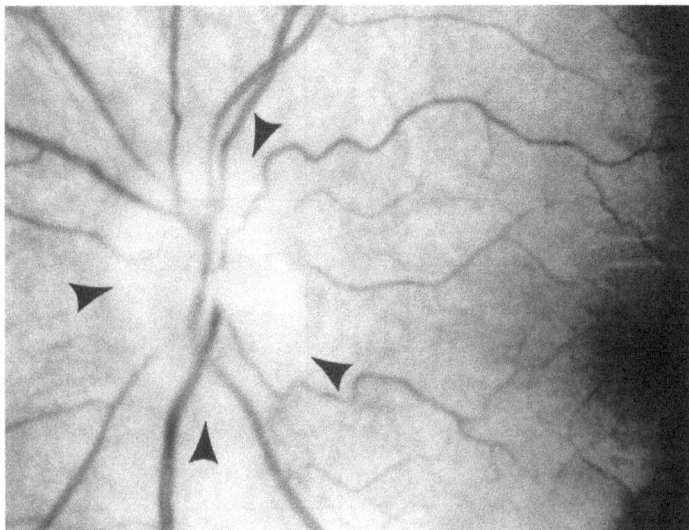

Fig. 12-4 Partial resolution of papilledema in the left eye 24 days after treatment with prednisone and acetazolamide (Diamox). Same magnification as in Figure 12-1. Arrowheads outline extent of disc edema.

acetazolamide (Diamox), 500 mg twice per day, was substituted for methazolamide (Neptazane), 50 mg three times daily. When seen again 6 weeks later, the patient's visual acuity had returned to 20/20 OU. She identified 11 Ishihara color plates with each eye. The paracentral scotoma had disappeared in the right eye and the field defect in the left eye had improved (mean sensitivity 26.3 dB) (Figure 12-3). Papilledema was significantly improved (Figure 12-4).

Comment

This case illustrates that PTC is a chronic disease with potential for recurrence in about 20% of patients. When treated aggressively, PTC can often can be managed effectively with pharmacotherapy.

REFERENCES

1. Radhakrishnan K, Ahlskog JE, Garrity JA, et al. Idiopathic intracranial hypertension. Mayo Clin Proc 1994;69:169.
2. Tomsak RL, Sweeney PJ. Pseudotumor cerebri: some neuro-ophthalmologic perspectives. In Daroff RB, Conomy JP (eds), Contributions to Contemporary Neurology: A Tribute to Joseph M. Foley. Stoneham, MA: Butterworth, 1988;201.
3. King JO, Mitchell PJ, Thomson KR, et al. Cerebral venography and manometry in idiopathic intracranial hypertension. Neurology 1995;45:2224.
4. Corbett JJ, Digre K. Idiopathic intracranial hypertension. An answer to, "the chicken or the egg"? Neurology 2002;58:5.
5. Selhorst JB, Waybright EA, Jennings S, et al. Liver lover's headache: pseudotumor cerebri and vitamin A intoxication. JAMA 1984;252:3365.
6. Gardner K, Cox T, Digre KB. Idiopathic intracranial hypertension associated with tetracycline use in fraternal twins: case reports and review. Neurology 1995;45:6.
7. Chiu AM, Chuenkongkaew WL, Cornblath WT, et al. Minocycline treatment and pseudotumor cerebri syndrome. Am J Ophthalmol 1998;126:116.
8. Lee AG, Golnik K, Kardon R, et al. Sleep apnea and intracranial hypertension in men. Ophthalmology 2002;109:482.
9. Purvin VA, Trobe JD, Kosmorsky G. Neuro-ophthalmic features of cerebral venous obstruction. Arch Neurol 1995;52:880.
10. King JO, Mitchell PJ, Thomson KR, Tress BM. Manometry combined with cervical puncture in idiopathic intracranial hypertension. Neurology 2002;58:26.
11. Scott IU, Siatkowski RM, Eneyni M, et al. Idiopathic intracranial hypertension in children and adolescents. Am J Ophthalmol 1997;124:253.
12. Cinciripini GS, Donahue S, Borchert MS. Idiopathic intracranial hypertension in prepubertal pediatric patients: characteristics, treatment, and outcome. Am J Ophthalmol 1999;127:178.
13. Sugerman HJ, Felton III WL, Salvant JB Jr, et al. Effects of surgically induced weight loss on idiopathic intracranial hypertension in morbid obesity. Neurology 1995;45:1655.
14. Sugerman HJ, Felton WL, Sismanis A, et al. Gastric surgery for pseudotumor cerebri associated with severe obesity. Ann Surg 1999;229:634.
15. Digre KB, Corbett JJ. Pseudotumor cerebri in men. Arch Neurol 1988;45:866.
16. Friedman DI, Rausch EA. Headache diagnoses in patients with treated idiopathic intracranial hypertension. Neurology 2002;58:1551.
17. Raskin NH. Headache (2nd ed). New York: Churchill Livingstone, 1988;289.
18. Wall M. Idiopathic intracranial hypertension: mechanisms of visual loss and disease management. Sem Neurol 2000;20:89.
19. Pollack S. Acute papilledema and visual loss in a patient with pseudotumor cerebri. Arch Ophthalmol 1987;105:752.

20. Gittinger JW, Asdourian GK. Macular abnormalities in papilledema from pseudotumor cerebri. Ophthalmology 1989;96:192.
21. Jacobson DM. Intracranial hypertension and the syndrome of acquired hyperopia with choroidal folds. J Neuroophthalmol 1995;15:178.
22. Krishna R, Kosmorsky GS, Wright KW. Pseudotumor cerebri sine papilledema with unilateral sixth nerve palsy. J Neuro-ophthalmol 1998;18:53.
23. Quattrone A, Bono F, Oliveri RL, et al. Cerebral venous thrombosis and isolated intracranial hypertension without papilledema in CDH. Neurology 2001;57:31.
24. Wall M, George D. Idiopathic intracranial hypertension (pseudotumor cerebri): a prospective study of 50 patients. Brain 1991;114:155.
25. Wall M, George D. Visual loss in pseudotumor cerebri: incidence and defects related to visual field strategy. Arch Neurol 1987;44:170.
26. Corbett JJ, Savino PJ, Thompson HS, et al. Visual loss in pseudotumor cerebri: follow-up of 57 patients from five to 41 years and a profile of 14 patients with permanent severe visual loss. Arch Neurol 1982;39:461.
27. Orcutt JC, Page NGR, Sanders MD. Factors affecting visual loss in benign intracranial hypertension. Ophthalmology 1984;91:1303.
28. Corbett JJ. Problems in the diagnosis and treatment of pseudotumor cerebri. Can J Neurol Sci 1983;10:221.
29. Speer C, Pearlman J, Phillips PH, et al. Fourth cranial nerve palsy in pediatric patients with pseudotumor cerebri. Am J Ophthalmol 1999;127:236.
30. Zachariah SB, Jimenez L, Zachariah B, et al. Pseudotumor cerebri with focal neurological deficit. J Neurol Neurosurg Psychiatry 1990;53:360.
31. Friedman DI, Jacobson DM. Diagnostic criteria for idiopathic intracranial hypertension. Neurology 2002;59:1492.
32. Brodsky MC, Vaphiades M. Magnetic resonance imaging in pseudotumor cerebri. Ophthalmol 1998;105:1696.
33. Cohen SM, Keltner JL. Thrombosis of the lateral transverse sinus with papilledema. Arch Ophthalmol 1993;111:275.
34. Lee AG, Brazis PW. Magnetic resonance venography in idiopathic pseudotumor cerebri. J Neuro-ophthalmol 2000;20:12.
35. Verplanck M, Kaufman DI, Parsons T, et al. Electrophysiology versus psychophysics in the detection of visual loss in pseudotumor cerebri. Neurology 1988;38:1789.
36. Lichter PR. Reducing side effects of carbonic anhydrase inhibitors. Ophthalmology 1981;88:266.
37. Tomsak RL, Niffenegger AS, Remler BF. Treatment of pseudotumor cerebri with Diamox (acetazolamide). J Clin Neuroophthalmol 1988;8:93.
38. Fishman RA. Cerebrospinal Fluid in Diseases of the Nervous System, 2nd ed. Philadelphia: Saunders, 1992.
39. Pagan FL, Restrepo L, Balish M, et al. A new drug for an old condition? Headache 2002;42;695.
40. Liu GT, Glaser JS, Schatz NJ. High-dose methylprednisolone and acetazolamide for visual loss in pseudotumor cerebri. Am J Ophthalmol 1994;118:88.
41. Goodwin JA. Treatment of idiopathic intracranial hypertension with digoxin. Ann Neurol 1990;28:248.
42. Newborg B. Pseudotumor cerebri treated by rice/reduction diet. Arch Intern Med 1974;133:802.
43. Johnson LN, Krohel GB, Madsen RW, March GA. The role of weight loss and acetazolamide in the treatment of idiopathic intracranial hypertension (pseudotumor cerebri). Ophthalmol 1998;105:2313.
44. Dandy WE. Intracranial pressure without brain tumor: diagnosis and treatment. Ann Surg 1937:106:492.
45. Bret P, Huppert J, Massini B, et al. Lumbar peritoneal shunt in non-hydrocephalic patients: a review of 41 cases. Acta Neurochir (Wein) 1986;80:90.

46. Rosenberg ML, Corbett JJ, Smith C, et al. Cerebrospinal fluid diversion procedures in pseudotumor cerebri. Neurology 1993;43:1071.
47. Eggenberger ER, Miller NR, Vitale S. Lumboperitoneal shunt for the treatment of pseudotumor cerebri. Neurology 1996;46:1524.
48. Burgett RA, Purvin VA, Kawasaki A. Lumboperitoneal shunting for pseudotumor cerebri. Neurology 1997;49:734.
49. Flaharty PM, Sergott RC. Optic nerve sheath decompression. Ophthalmol Clin North America 1992;5:395.
50. Kersten RC, Kulwin DR. Optic nerve sheath fenestration through a lateral canthotomy incision. Arch Ophthalmol 1993;111:870.
51. Spoor TC, McHenry JG, Shin DH. Optic nerve sheath decompression with adjunctive mitomycin and Molteno device implantation. Arch Ophthalmol 1994;112:25.
52. Spoor TC, Ramocki JM, Madion MP, et al. Treatment of pseudotumor cerebri by primary and secondary optic nerve sheath decompression. Am J Ophthalmol 1991;112:177.
53. Kelman SE, Heaps R, Wolf A, et al. Optic nerve decompression surgery improves visual function in patients with pseudotumor cerebri. Neurosurgery 1992;30:391.
54. Banta JT, Farris BK. Pseudotumor cerebri and optic nerve sheath decompression. Ophthalmology 2000;107;1907.
55. Mauriello JA, Shaderowfsky P, Gizzi M, et al. Management of visual loss after optic nerve sheath decompression in patients with pseudotumor cerebri. Ophthalmology 1995;102:441.
56. Jacobson EE, Johnston IH, McCluskey P. The effect of optic nerve sheath decompression on CSF dynamics in pseudotumor cerebri and related conditions. J Clin Neurosci 1999;375.
57. Hayreh SS. Pathogenesis of oedema of the optic disc. Doc Ophthalmol 1968;24:289.
58. Kaye AH, Galbraith JEK, King J. Intracranial pressure following optic nerve decompression for benign intracranial hypertension. J Neurosurg 1981;55:453.
59. Villain M, Sandillon F, Muller A, et al. Macroglial alterations after isolated optic nerve sheath fenestration in rabbit. Invest Ophthalmol Vis Sci 2002;43:120.
60. Mittra RA, Sergott RC, Flaharty PM, et al. Optic nerve decompression improves hemodynamic parameters in papilledema. Ophthalmology 1993;100:987.
61. Seiff SR, Shah L. A model for the mechanism of optic nerve sheath fenestration. Arch Ophthalmol 1990;108:1326.
62. Kelman SE, Sergott RC, Cioffi GA, et al. Modified optic nerve decompression in patients with functioning lumboperitoneal shunts and progressive visual loss. Ophthalmology 1991;98:1449.
63. Sergott RC, Savino PJ, Bosley TM. Optic nerve sheath decompression: a clinical review and proposed pathophsiologic mechanism. Aust NZ J Ophthalmol 1990;18:365.
64. Flynn WJ, Westfall CT, Weisman JS. Transient blindness after optic nerve sheath fenestration. Am J Opthalmol 1994;117:678.
65. Nicholas J, Higgins P, Owler BK, Cousins C, Pickard JD. Venous sinus stenting for refractory benign intracranial hypertension. Lancet 2002;359:228.

13

Retinal Artery Occlusion

OVERVIEW AND ETIOLOGY

Central retinal artery occlusion (CRAO) is a devastating ocular event with a dismal visual prognosis. Men are affected somewhat more than women. Between 30% and 77% of patients suffering a CRAO have hypertensive or atherosclerotic cardiovascular disease. Two percent to 17% have cardiac valvular disease. More than three fourths have significant carotid artery disease as demonstrated by carotid angiography [1]. Patients tend to be in their sixth and seventh decades and, in up to 50%, CRAO is their first neurovascular symptom. Depending on the series, CRAO occurs as a result of coronary artery surgery, carotid endarterectomy, or carotid angiography in approximately 25%. Patients younger than 40 years of age with CRAO often have vasculitis, cardiac valve disease, or are in a hypercoagulable state [1-4]. Some unusual presentations of CRAO are listed in Table 13-1 [5-10].

Branch retinal artery occlusions (BRAOs) occur in the patient population with the same risk factors for CRAO. Additionally, there are a number of other diseases, especially in young adults, that have BRAO as a manifestation (Table 13-2) [3,4,11-17].

CLINICAL SIGNS AND SYMPTOMS

The clinical presentation of CRAO is described in Box 13-1 (see also Figure 13-1). In some patients with CRAO, a cilioretinal artery, arising from the choroidal circulation, spares a portion of the retina from infarction. Conversely, isolated cilioretinal artery occlusion can occur [18].

Aftereffects of CRAO include optic atrophy, secondary glaucoma, and optic disc neovascularization. An unusual form of the latter has been called circumpapillary cilioretinal anastomoses or "Nettleship

Table 13-1   Some Unusual Presentations of Central Retinal Artery Occlusion

Presentation	Reference
Migrainous CRAO	5
As part of radiation retinopathy	6
Relapsing-remitting or chronic CRAO	7,8
From cocaine abuse	9
Following varicella infection	10
From temporal arteritis (see Chapter 14)	

CRAO = central retinal artery occlusion.

Table 13-2 Some Other Presentations of Branch Retinal Artery Occlusion	
Presentation	Reference
Idiopathic recurrent branch retinal artery occlusion	11,12
Coronary angioplasty	13
Multifocal retinitis and cat scratch disease	14
Systemic lupus erythematosus	3
Subacute bacterial endocarditis	3
Antiphospholipid antibody syndrome	3,4
Acute myelogenous leukemia	3
Behçet's disease	3
Protein S deficiency	3
Oral contraceptive use	3
Migraine	3
Mitral valve papillary elastoma	15
Microangiopathy of the brain, retina, and ear in young women (Susac's syndrome)	16
Dissection of internal carotid artery	29

collaterals" [19]. The most important sequelae of CRAO, however, are hemispheric stroke or cardiovascular death.

Branch retinal artery occlusion is much like CRAO. However, because less of the retina is affected, vision loss is not as severe as with CRAO (Figure 13-2).

Both CRAO and BRAO may be heralded by transient monocular blindness (see Chapter 16).

INVESTIGATIONS

The evaluation of CRAO and BRAO is similar to that outlined for transient monocular blindness (see Chapter 16). In younger patients with CRAO or BRAO, more attention needs to be paid to the possibility of cardiogenic emboli, vasculitis, and hypercoagulable states [20].

TREATMENT

Treatments for CRAO and BRAO are rarely effective, even if the patient is seen within hours of vision loss [21-24]. Table 13-3 [2,19,21-30] lists a variety of approaches that may be tried.

Box 13-1   Signs and Symptoms of Central Retinal Artery Occlusion
Sudden, painless loss of vision to counting fingers or less
Relative afferent pupillary defect
Severe visual field loss
Fundus shows arteriolar narrowing, segmentation of blood column, opacification of retina, and macular "cherry red spot"
Emboli may or may not be seen
Retinal hemorrhages are rare

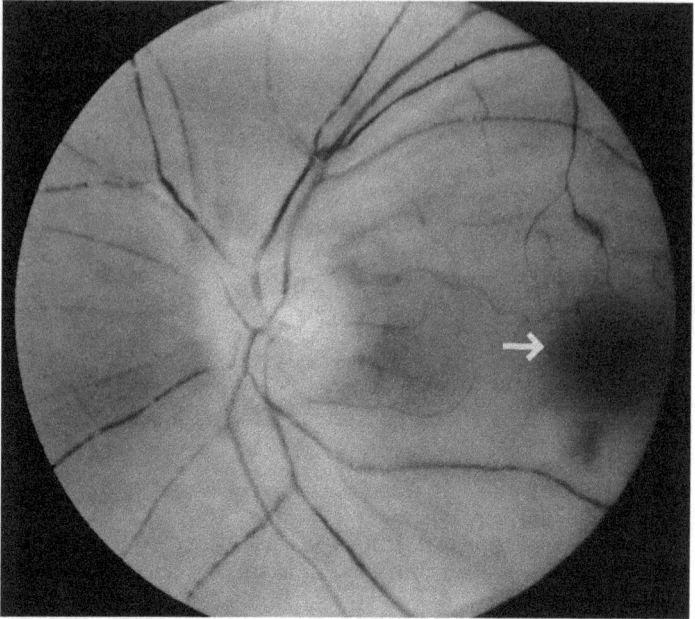

Fig. 13-1 Central retinal artery occlusion in the left eye. The blood column is segmented in both retinal arteries and veins from sluggish flow. The retina has lost its transparency from ischemia. Dark area to right *(arrow)* would appear as a "cherry red spot " in a color photograph corresponding to oxygenated blood in the choroid seen through the thinner foveal retina.

If the patient has impairment in retinal perfusion at the time of the initial examination, with evidence of segmentation of the arterial blood column and very low retinal artery pressure,* my (RT) preferred treatment is anterior chamber paracentesis to quickly lower intraocular pressure to zero in the hopes of raising retinal perfusion pressure. If retinal perfusion has been restored by the time the patient is first seen, invasive procedures are of little use. The exceptions would be a chronic partial retinal artery occlusion [8] or venous stasis retinopathy [31]. If there is any chance that temporal arteritis is the cause of CRAO or BRAO, the use of high-dose systemic steroids is mandatory (see Chapter 14).

Other treatments are individualized on a case-by-case basis. The newest approach is local intraarterial fibrinolysis. However, the number of studies evaluating this technique are small and a center using "brain attack" protocols must be reached within a few hours for the technique to be effective [29,30].

---

*See Chapter 16, Transient Monocular Blindness, for a method of estimating retinal artery pressure.

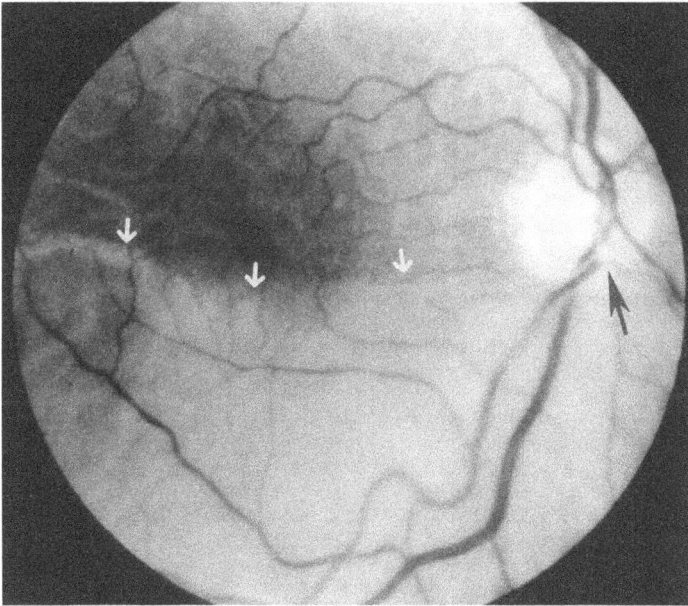

Fig. 13-2 Embolic branch retinal artery occlusion in the right eye. An embolus (*black arrow*) can be seen at the first bifurcation of the inferior temporal branch artery. The inferior retina has become ischemic and the demarcation line is indicated by the *white arrows*.

Table 13-3 Treatments for Central and Branch Retinal Artery Occlusion

Treatment	Reference
Ocular massage	2,21,22
Inhalation of 5% carbon dioxide, 95% oxygen	25
Retrobulbar injection of lidocaine (Xylocaine) papaverine, or aminophylline	2
Anterior chamber paracentesis	20,25
Acetazolamide (Diamox)	2,20
Anticoagulation	20,26
Thrombolytic therapy	27,28,30,31
Retrograde perfusion of the central retinal artery with heparin and papaverine after cannulation of the supraorbital artery	2,28
Steroids and other immunosuppressants	18,20
Sublingual isosorbide dinitrate	20
Calcium channel blockers (see Chapter 16)	
Hyperbaric oxygen	22

Whenever possible, the exact etiology of the retinal artery occlusion should be identified to prevent other attacks of ischemia to the eye, brain, or other organs [32].

REFERENCES

1. Tomsak RL, Hanson M, Gutman FA. Carotid artery disease and central retinal artery occlusion. Cleve Clin Q 1979;46:7.
2. Tomsak RL, Ross D, Gutman FA. Central retinal artery occlusion. Perspect Ophthalmol 1978;2:217.
3. Greven CM, Slusher MM, Weaver RG. Retinal arterial occlusions in young adults. Am J Ophthalmol 1995;120:776.
4. Dori D, Beiran I, Gelfand Y, et al. Multiple retinal arteriolar occlusions associated with coexisting primary antiphospholipid syndrome and factor V Leiden mutation. Am J Ophthalmol 2000;129:106.
5. Katz B. Migrainous central retinal artery occlusion. J Clin Neuroophthalmol 1986;6;69.
6. Noble KG. Central retinal artery occlusion: the presenting sign in radiation retinopathy. Arch Ophthalmol 1994;112:1409.
7. Werner MS, Latchaw R, Baker L, et al. Relapsing and remitting central retinal artery occlusion. Am J Ophthalmol 1994;118:393.
8. Perkins SA, Magargal LE, Augsburger JJ, et al. The idling retina: reversible visual loss in central retinal artery obstruction. Ann Ophthalmol 1987;19:3.
9. Sleiman I, Mangili R, Semeraro F, et al. Cocaine-associated retinal vascular occlusion: report of two cases. Am J Med 1994;97:198.
10. Cho N-C, Han H-J. Central retinal artery occlusion after varicella. Am J Ophthalmol 1992;113:591.
11. Johnson MW, Flynn HW, Gass JDM. Idiopathic recurrent branch retinal arterial occlusion. Arch Ophthalmol 1989;107:757.
12. Johnson MW, Thomley ML, Huang S, et al. Idiopathic recurrent branch retinal arterial occlusion. Natural history and laboratory evaluation. Ophthalmology 1994;101:480.
13. Filatov V, Tom D, Alexandrakis G, et al. Branch retinal artery occlusion associated with directional coronary atherectomy after percutaneous transluminal coronary angioplasty. Am J Ophthalmol 1995;120:391.
14. Cohen SM, Davis JL, Gass JDM. Branch retinal arterial occlusions in multifocal retinitis with optic nerve edema. Arch Ophthalmol 1995;113:1271.
15. Zamora RL, Adelberg DA, Berger AS, et al. Branch retinal artery occlusion caused by a mitral valve papillary fibroelastoma. Am J Ophthalmol 1995;119:325.
16. Susac JO. Susac's syndrome: the triad of microangiopathy of the brain and retina with hearing loss in young women. Neurology 1994;44:591.
17. McDonough RL, Forteza AM, Flynn, Jr HW. Internal carotid artery dissection causing a branch retinal artery occlusion in a young adult. Am J Ophthalmol 1998;125:704-06.
18. Horton JC. Embolic cilioretinal artery occlusion with atherosclerosis of the ipsilateral carotid artery. Retina 1995;15:441.
19. Ragge NK, Hoyt WF. Nettleship collaterals: circumpapillary cilioretinal anastomoses after occlusion of the central retinal artery. Br J Ophthalmol 1992;76:186.
20. Perler BA. Hypercoagulability and the hypercoagulability syndromes. Am J Radiol 1995;164:559.
21. Rumelt S, Dorenboim Y, Rehany U. Aggressive systematic treatment for central retinal artery occlusion. Am J Ophthalmol 1999;128:733.
22. Schmidt D. Ocular massage in a case of central retinal artery occlusion: the successful treatment of a hitherto undescribed type of embolism. Eur J Med Res 2000;5:157.
23. Aisenbrey S, Krott R, Heller R, et al. Hyperbaric oxygen therapy in retinal artery occlusion. Ophthalmologe 2000;97:461. (in German).
24. Fraser S, Siriwardena D. Interventions for non-arteritic central retinal artery occlusion (Cochrane Review). In: The Cochrane Library, Issue 2002. Oxford: Update Software.

25. Atebara NH, Brown GC, Cater J. Efficacy of anterior chamber paracentesis and carbogen in treating acute nonarteritic central retinal artery occlusion. Ophthalmology 1995;102:2029.
26. Becker RC, Ansell J. Antithrombotic therapy: an abbreviated reference for clinicians. Arch Intern Med 1995;155:149.
27. Mames RN, Shugar JK, Levey N, et al. Peripheral thrombolytic therapy for central retinal artery occlusion. Arch Ophthalmol 1995;113:1094.
28. Schmidt D, Adelman G. Is it feasible to use the supratrochlear artery for inducing intra-arterial fibrinolysis in cases of central retinal artery occlusion? Neuroophthalmology 1995;15:265.
29. Beatty S, Au Eong KG. Local intra-arterial fibrinolysis for acute occlusion of the central retinal artery: a meta-analysis of the published data. Br J Ophthalmol 2000;84:914.
30. Podolecchia R, Puglioli M, Ragone MC, et al. Superselective intraarterial fibrinolysis in central retinal artery occlusion. Am J Neuroradiol 1999;20:565.
31. Klijn CJ, Kappelle LJ, van Schooneveld MJ, et al. Venous stasis retinopathy in symptomatic carotid artery occlusion: prevalence, cause, and outcome. Stroke 2002;33:695.
32. Wong TY, Klein R, Cooper LS, et al. Retinal microvascular abnormalities and incident stroke: the Atherosclerosis Risk in Communities Study. Lancet 2001;358:1134.

14

Giant Cell (or Temporal) Arteritis

OVERVIEW AND ETIOLOGY

Temporal arteritis (TA; also called giant cell, or cranial, arteritis) is a vasculitis that usually affects the arteries of the head and neck of those in the geriatric age group. The mean age at presentation is 70 years. White women are affected somewhat more often than men and the disease is less common in blacks, Hispanics, and Asians [1-3]. The prevalence is higher in northern climates and in those of Scandinavian ancestry [4]. There may be a higher incidence in the fall and winter [2]. Familial cases are rare but have been reported [1]. Temporal arteritis is a chronic disease that may recur even if treated [5] and may be fatal [6]. The pathogenesis is immunologic, and the inflammatory response involves platelet-derived growth factors; interferon-gamma; macrophages; and interleukins 1, 2, and 6 [7,8]. Increased endothelin-1 levels may play a role in ischemic complications [9]. Atypical clinical presentations are well documented [10].

There is an overlap between polymyalgia rheumatica (PMR) and giant cell arteritis (GCA) in that between 16% and 21% of patients with PMR have a positive temporal artery biopsy result and 40-60% of persons with GCA have symptoms of PMR [8].

MAIN CLINICAL FEATURES

The main clinical features of TA are listed in Boxes 14-1 through 14-3 [11-14]. Occult giant cell arteritis presenting with visual signs or symptoms (e.g., biopsy-proven GCA with no systemic symptoms) is not uncommon [15]. Therefore, GCA should be in the differential diagnosis

---

Box 14-1   Ophthalmologic Manifestations of Temporal Arteritis

Anterior ischemic optic neuropathy (most common presentation)
Posterior ischemic optic neuropathy
Ischemic retinopathy, retinal, and cilioretinal artery occlusions
Amaurosis fugax
Diplopia
Ophthalmoplegia, ptosis, and miosis
Anterior segment ischemia
Marginal corneal ulceration
Uveitic glaucoma
Orbital apex syndrome
Tonic pupil
Eye pain

Box 14-2   Neurologic Manifestations of Temporal Arteritis

Headache
Neuropathies
Transient ischemic attacks/strokes
Neuro-otologic syndromes (e.g., lingual infarction)
Tremor
Neuropsychiatric syndromes (e.g., depression, visual hallucinations)
Myelopathy

Box 14-3   Systemic Manifestations of Temporal Arteritis Commonly Associated with Positive Biopsy Results

Fatigue
Weight loss
Fever
Jaw claudication
Temporal artery tenderness
Polymyalgia rheumatica

of anyone older than 55 years of age who presents with any of the conditions listed in Box 14-1.

INVESTIGATIONS
Blood Tests

A number of laboratory tests have been used to aid in the diagnosis and management of TA. Some of the more common tests are listed in Box 14-4.

Although the Westergren sedimentation rate is most commonly used because of its sensitivity, it is a very nonspecific test [16-18]. In my (RT) experience, testing for plasma fibrinogen concentration is more useful for diagnosing and following disease activity in TA because of its well-defined upper and lower limits of normality (200-400 mg%), and because, in most cases, the sedimentation rate is predominantly determined by plasma fibrinogen concentration [19] (Figure 14-1). Afshari and colleagues also recommend plasma fibrinogen determination as an adjunctive diagnostic test for GCA [20]. Furthermore, recent literature has shown that plasma fibrinogen concentration, in itself, is a risk factor for ischemic events [21-26]. See Box 14-5 for a list of drugs that lower fibrinogen concentration.

Box 14-4   Laboratory Tests in Temporal Arteritis

Westergren sedimentation rate
Temporal artery biopsy
Fibrinogen
C-reactive protein
Platelet count (elevated)
von Willebrand factor
Serum alkaline phosphatase
Serum aspartate amino transferase
Anticardiolipin antibodies

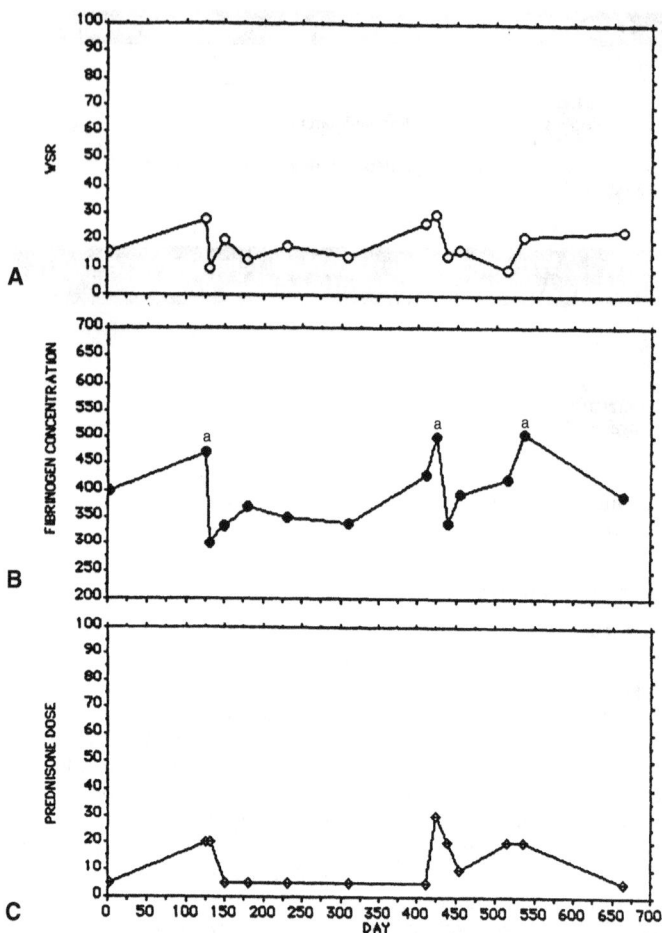

Fig. 14-1 Test results for a 68-year-old female with anterior ischemic optic neuropathy in the right eye and positive terminal artery biopsy followed for almost 2 years. A. Sequential Westergren sedimentation rates; B. simultaneous fibrinogen determinations; C. Prednisone dose. Episodes of clinical exacerbation of disease activity are indicated by *a*. Note that Westergren sedimentation rates do not exceed 30 mm/hour, whereas elevation in fibrinogen concentration (>400 mg%) accompanied return of symptoms.

Hayreh and colleagues [27] have shown the use of elevated C-reactive protein in diagnosing GCA. A C-reactive protein value above 2.45 mg/dl in association with a Westergren sedimentation rate of 47 mm/hr or more provided 97% specificity in diagnosis of GCA.

Antiphospholipid antibodies are elevated in GCA [28,29] and levels seem to parallel disease activity [29].

Thrombocytosis has proved useful for diagnosis of GCA in the hands of various investigators [30-32]. Platelet count of 400,000 or greater was correlated with a positive temporal artery biopsy result by Foroozan and colleagues [32].

Given the above, my general routine is to order the following initial tests in a patient suspected of having TA: complete blood cell count, including platelets; fibrinogen; C-reactive protein; and Westergren sedimentation rate. Note that C-reactive protein levels rise within hours after an inflammatory stimulus, fibrinogen levels peak about 2 weeks later, and thrombocytosis takes months to manifest itself in the setting of GCA [31,33]. I base the need for a temporal artery biopsy on the lab values in combination with clinical symptoms (see Boxes 14-1 to 14-3). Whenever possible, the aid of a rheumatologist is enlisted for management after the diagnosis is made.

Temporal Artery Biopsy

A simple method for performing a temporal artery biopsy is given by Tomsak [34]. The classic histologic picture of TA (Figure 14-2) is marked

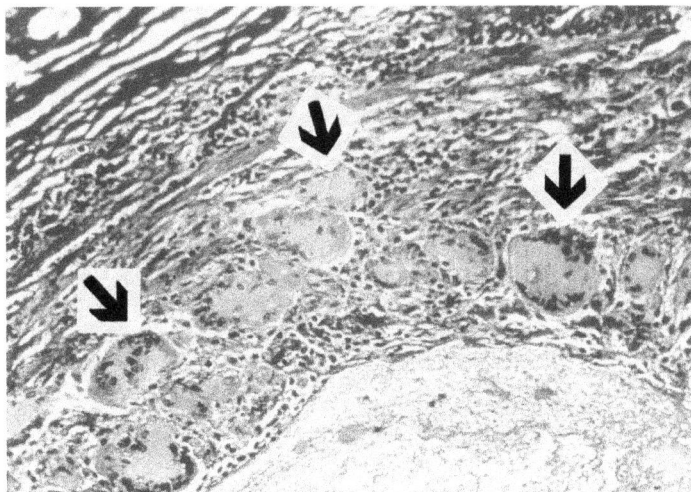

Fig. 14-2 Positive temporal artery biopsy result. Arrows point to giant cells.

by intimal thickening and destruction of the internal elastic lamina (99% prevalence) associated with dense granulomatous inflammation including lymphocytes, histiocytes and giant cells (66% prevalence), and fibrinoid necrosis (12% prevalence) [35,36]. Healed arteritis is characterized by fragmented and lost internal elastic lamina, medial fibrosis, and adventitial scarring [35], although the ability to diagnose healed arteritis is controversial [37]. Combining data from 20 reports totalling 2,680 patients, the overall positivity rate for temporal artery biopsies is 39% [38].

How large should a biopsy specimen be? Chambers and Bernardino [39] showed that a biopsy as small as 4 mm, if serially sectioned meticulously, results in a false-negative result rate of less than 1%. Another report showed that multiple sectioning improved the yield of positive biopsy results by 8.9%, but concluded that the extra work needed was not cost effective! [40]. Skip areas do exist [41,42], and false-negative biopsy results have been reported with incidences from 5 to 61% [35]. These conflicting statistics highlight the importance of the pathologist's role in the diagnosis of TA [43].

Can a temporal artery biopsy be performed after beginning steroid treatment? A common myth regarding TA is that the biopsy must be performed before systemic steroid treatment. This clinical approach invites visual and medicolegal disasters. For example, Achkar and co-workers [44] found that the positivity rate of temporal artery biopsies was unrelated to previous corticosteroid treatment in a series of 535 patients. To and colleagues [45] found a positive biopsy result in a woman who had been taking 60 mg of prednisone a day for $4\frac{1}{2}$ weeks. Evans and colleagues [46] documented active arteritis at autopsy in a man who died of an unrelated coronary occlusion, with TA treated with steroids for 6 weeks, and similar results were obtained by Ray-Chaudhuri and co-workers in six patients [47].

Therefore, steroid therapy must be begun immediately in any case of suspected TA, and the biopsy should be scheduled in a timely, but nonemergent, fashion. In selected cases, repeat temporal artery biopsies are indicated [48,42]. Bilateral simultaneous biopsies increase the diagnostic yield by approximately 3% [49,50].

Ultrasound

Color duplex ultrasonography has been applied to the superficial temporal artery in those suspected of having GCA [51]. The presence of a dark halo around segments of the artery seems to correlate well with biopsy positivity. In another study, tenderness of the artery to palpation was more useful than ultrasonography in predicting a positive biopsy result [52].

Intravenous Fluorescein Angiography

Choroidal filling defects have been demonstrated by intravenous fluorescein angiography (IVFA) in anterior ischemic optic neuropathy (AION) caused by giant cell arteritis, but not in the nonarteritic variety of AION [53,54]. Indocyanine green angiography does not add useful information to that provided by IVFA [55].

TREATMENT
Corticosteroids
Oral prednisone, in a daily dose (not alternate day) of a least 40 mg, must be given [56]. Intravenous methylprednisolone, 250-500 mg four times a day, has been advocated for patients with acute vision loss from TA [57], but even this approach may not be protective of progressive vision loss [58-60]. Furthermore, aggressive treatment with intravenous steroids only improves vision loss approximately 4% of the time [61] and does not seem to have a long-term steroid-sparing effect [62]. Remember that chronic steroid use can cause hypertension, diabetes mellitus, osteoporosis, compression fractures, myopathy, and so forth [63,64]. Complications occur twice as often in patients older than 75 years of age. Side effects are dose-related and more frequent in those started on prednisone, 40 mg per day or greater. Patients who present with symptoms of a strong inflammatory response — fever, weight loss, sedimentation rate greater than 85 mm/hr, and anemia — require higher initial doses of corticosteroids and a longer duration of therapy [65].

Other
Dapsone [66] and methotrexate [8,67] have also been used in selected cases, but the usefulness of methotrexate as a steroid-sparing agent in giant cell arteritis has been questioned recently after a large multicenter study [68]. Infliximab, an antitumor necrosis factor, may be an alternative treatment in steroid-resistant cases of GCA [69].

CLINICAL COURSE AND PROGNOSIS
Paulley and Hughes [70] stated that "giant cell arteritis, once believed to run a benign course, kills or maims a number of those affected, and when in remission, it may only sleep." As an example of this behavior, Blumberg and others [5] reported the case of an elderly woman with biopsy-proven disease in whom, 9 years later, recurrent clinical symptoms developed; repeat biopsy results were again positive for acute TA. Thus, TA is a chronic disease that requires periodic monitoring of symptoms and laboratory values.

REFERENCES
1. Fietta P, Manganelli P, Zanetti A, Neri TM. Familial giant cell arteritis and polymyalgia rheumatica: aggregation in 2 families. J Rheumatol 2002;29:1551.
2. Petursdottir V, Johansson H, Nordborg E, Nordborg C. The epidemiology of biopsy-positive giant cell arteritis: special reference to cyclic fluctuations. Rheumatology 1999;38:1208.
3. Grosser SJ, Reddy RK, Tomsak RL, Katzin WE. Temporal arteritis in African Americans. Neuro-ophthalmol 1999;21:25.

4. Liu NH, LaBree LD, Feldon SE, Rao NA. The epidemiology of giant cell arteritis: a 12-year retrospective study. Ophthalmology 2001;108:1145.

5. Blumberg S, Giansiracusa DF, Docken WP, et al. Recurrence of temporal arteritis: clinical recurrence nine years after initial illness. JAMA 1980;244:1713.

6. Save-Soderbergh J, Malmvall B-O, Andersson R, et al. Giant cell arteritis as a cause of death: report of nine cases. JAMA 1986;255:493.

7. Kaiser M, Weyand CM, Bjornsson J, Goronzy JJ. Platelet-derived growth factor, intimal hyperplasia, and ischemic complications in giant cell arteritis. Arthritis Rheum 1998;41:623.

8. Salvarani C, Cantini F, Boiardi L, Hunder GG. Polymyalgia rheumatica and giant-cell arteritis. N Engl J Med 2002;347:261.

9. Pache M, Kaiser HJ, Haufschild T, et al. Increased endothelin-1 plasma levels in giant cell arteritis: a report on four patients. Am J Ophthalmol 2002;133:160.

10. Strachan RW, How J, Bewsher PD. Masked giant-cell arteritis. Lancet 1980;l:194.

11. Hayreh SS, Podhajsky PA, Zimmerman B. Ocular manifestations of giant cell arteritis. Am J Ophthalmol 1998;125:509.

12. Tang RA. Giant cell arteritis diagnosis and management. Semin Ophthalmol 1988;3:244.

13. Gonzalez-Gay MA, Blanco R, Rodriguez-Valverde V, et al. Permanent visual loss and cerebrovascular accidents in giant cell arteritis: predictors and response to treatment. Arthritis Rheum 1998;41:1497.

14. Semmler A, Urbach H, Klockgether T. Giant cell arteritis causing multiple vertebro-basilar infarcts. Neurology 2002;58:1399.

15. Hayreh SS, Podhajsky PA, Zimmerman B. Occult giant cell arteritis: ocular manifestations. Am J Ophthalmol 1998;125:521.

16. Sox HC, Liang MH. The erythrocyte sedimentation rate: guidelines for rational use. Ann Intern Med 1986;104:515.

17. Jacobson DM, Slamovits TL. Erythrocyte sedimentation rate and its relationship to hematocrit in giant cell arteritis. Arch Ophthalmol 1987;105:965.

18. Weinstein A, Del Giudice J. The erythrocyte sedimentation rate-time honored and tradition bound. J Rheumatol 1994;21:1177.

19. Gudmundsson M, Nordborg E, Bengtsson B-A, et al. Plasma viscosity in giant cell arteritis as a predictor of disease activity. Ann Rheum Dis 1993;52:104.

20. Afshari NA, Afshari MA, Lessell S. Temporal arteritis. Int Ophthalmol Clin 2001;41:151.

21. Kannel WB, Wolf PA, Castelli WP, et al. Fibrinogen and risk of cardiovascular disease. The Framingham study. JAMA 1987;258:1183.

22. Somer T, Meiselman HJ. Disorders of blood viscosity. Ann Med 1993;25:31.

23. Clark WM, Coull BM, Beamer NB. Need for treatment of elevated plasma fibrinogen levels in cerebrovascular disease. Heart Dis Stroke 1993;2:503.

24. Folsom AR, Qamhieh HT, Flack JM, et al. Plasma fibrinogen: levels and correlates in young adults. Am J Epidemiol 1993;138:1023.

25. Eber B, Schumacher M. Fibrinogen: its role in the hemostatic regulation in atherosclerosis. Semin Thromb Hemost 1993;19:104.

26. Ernst E. Fibrinogen-an important risk factor for atherothrombotic diseases. Ann Med 1994;26:15.

27. Hayreh SS, Podhajsky PA, Raman R, Zimmerman B. Giant cell arteritis: validity and reliability of various diagnostic criteria. Am J Ophthalmol 1997;123:285.

28. Espinosa G, Tassies D, Font J, et al. Antiphospholipid antibodies and thrombophilic factors in giant cell arteritis. Semin Arthritis Rheum 2001;31:12.

29. Liozon E, Roblot P, Paire D, et al. Anticardiolipin antibody levels predict flares and relapses in patients with giant-cell (temporal) arteritis. Rheumatology 2000;39:1089.

30. Lincoff NS, Erlich PD, Brass LS. Thrombocytosis in temporal arteritis. Rising platelet counts: a red flag for giant cell arteritis. J Neuro-ophthalmol 2000;20:67.
31. Gonzalez-Alegre P, Ruiz-Lopez AD, Abarca-Costalago M, Gonzalez-Santos P. Increment of the platelet count in temporal arteritis: response to therapy and ischemic complications. Eur Neurol 2001;45:43.
32. Foroozan R, Danesh-Meyer H, Savino PJ, et al. Thrombocytosis in patients with biopsy-proven giant cell arteritis. Ophthalmology 2002;109:1267.
33. Gabay C, Kushner I. Acute-phase proteins and other systemic responses to inflammation. N Engl J Med 1999;340:448.
34. Tomsak RL. Superficial temporal artery biopsy: a simplified technique. J Clin Neuroophthalmol 1991;11:202.
35. McDonnell PJ, Moore GW, Miller NR, et al. Temporal arteritis: a clinicopathologic study. Ophthalmology 1986;93:518.
36. Baldursson O, Steinsson K, Bjornsson J, et al. Giant cell arteritis in Iceland – an epidemiologic and histopathologic analysis. Arthritis Rheum 1994;37:1007.
37. Cox M, Gilks B. Healed or quiescent temporal arteritis versus senescent changes in temporal artery biopsy specimens. Pathology 2001;33:163.
38. Smetana GW, Shmerling RH. Does this patient have temporal arteritis? JAMA 2002;287:92.
39. Chambers WA, Bernardino VB. Specimen length in temporal artery biopsies. J Clin Neuroophthalmol 1988;8:121.
40. Chakrabarty A, Franks AJ. Temporal artery biopsy: is there any value in examining biopsies at multiple levels? J Clin Pathol 2000;53:131.
41. Poller DN, van Wyk O, Jeffrey MJ. The importance of skip lesions in temporal arteritis. J Clin Pathol 2000;53:137.
42. Brownstein S, Nicolle DA, Codere F. Bilateral blindness in temporal arteritis with skip areas. Arch Ophthalmol 1983;101:388.
43. Fleming KA. Evidence-based cellular pathology. Lancet 2002;359:1149.
44. Achkar A A, Lie JT, Hunder GG, et al. How does previous corticosteroid treatment affect the biopsy findings in giant cell (temporal) arteritis? Ann Intern Med 1994;120:987.
45. To KW, Enzer YR, Tsiaras WG. Temporal artery biopsy after one month of corticosteroid therapy. Am J Ophthalmol 1994;117:265.
46. Evans JM, Batts KP, Hunder GG. Persistent giant cell arteritis despite corticosteroid treatment. Mayo Clin Proc 1994;69:1060.
47. Ray-Chaudhuri N, Kine DA, Tijani SO, et al. Effect of prior steroid treatment on temporal artery biopsy findings in giant cell arteritis. Br J Ophthalmol 2002;86:530.
48. Copetto JR, Montiero M. Diagnosis of highly occult giant cell arteritis by repeat temporal artery biopsies. Neuroophthalmology 1990; 10:217.
49. Boyev LR, Miller NR, Green WR. Efficacy of unilateral versus bilateral temporal artery biopsies for the diagnosis of giant cell arteritis. Am J Ophthalmol 1999;128:211.
50. Danesh-Meyer H, Savino PJ, Eagle RC, et al. Low diagnostic yield with second biopsies in suspected giant cell arteritis. J Neuro-ophthalmol 2000;20:213.
51. Schmidt WA, Keaft HE, Vorphal K, et al. Color duplex ultrasonography in the diagnosis of temporal arteritis. N Engl J Med 1997;337:1336.
52. Salvarani C, Silingardi M, Ghirarduzzi A, et al. Is duplex ultrasonography useful for the diagnosis of giant-cell arteritis? Ann Intern Med 2002;137:232.
53. Siatkowski RM, Gass JDM, Glaser JS, et al. Fluorescein angiography in the diagnosis of giant cell arteritis. Am J Ophthalmol 1993;115:57.
54. Arnold AC. Fluorescein angiographic characteristics of the optic disc in ischemic and glaucomatous optic neuropathy. Curr Opin Ophthalmol 1995;6:30.
55. Valmaggia C, Speiser P, Bischoff P, Niederberger H. Indocyanine green versus fluorescein angiography in the differential diagnosis of arteritic and nonarteritic anterior ischemic optic neuropathy. Retina 1999;19:131.

56. Hunder GG, Sheps SG, Alien GL, et al. Daily and alternate-day corticosteroid regimens in treatment of giant cell arteritis. Comparison in a prospective study. Ann Intern Med 1975;82:613.

57. Rosenfeld SI, Kosmorsky GS, Klingele TG, et al. Treatment of temporal arteritis with ocular involvement. Am J Med 1986;78:143.

58. Hwang JM, Girkin CA, Perry JD, et al. Bilateral ocular ischemic syndrome secondary to giant cell arteritis progressing despite corticosteroid treatment. Am J Ophthalmol 1999;127:102.

59. Staunton H, Stafford F, Leader M, O'Riordain D. Deterioration of giant cell arteritis with corticosteroid therapy. Arch Neurol 2000;57:581.

60. Slavin ML, Margolis AJ. Progressive anterior ischemic optic neuropathy due to giant cell arteritis despite high-dose intravenous corticosteroids [letter]. Arch Ophthalmol 1988;106:1167.

61. Hayreh SS, Zimmerman B, Kardon RH. Visual improvement with corticosteroid therapy in giant cell arteritis. Report of a large study and review of literature. Acta Ophthalmol Scand 2002;80:355.

62. Chevalet P, Barrier JH, Pottier P, et al. A randomized, multicenter controlled clinical trial using intravenous pulses of methylprednisolone in the initial treatment of simple forms of giant cell arteritis: a one year followup study of 164 patients. J Rheumatol 2000;27:1484.

63. Rubinow A, Brandt KD, Cohen AS, et al. Iatrogenic morbidity accompanying suppression of temporal arteritis by adrenal corticosteroids. Ann Ophthalmol 1984;16:258.

64. Nesher G, Sonnenblick M, Friedlander Y. Analysis of steroid related complications and mortality in temporal arteritis: a 15-year survey of 43 patients. J Rheumatol 1994;21:1283.

65. Hernandez-Rodriguez J, Garcia-Martinez A, Casademont J, et al. A strong initial systemic inflammatory response is associated with higher corticosteroid requirements and longer duration of therapy in patients with giant-cell arteritis. Arthritis Rheum 2002;47:29.

66. Reinitz E, Aversa A. Long-term treatment of temporal arteritis with dapsone. Am J Med 1988;85:456.

67. Wilke WS, Biro JA, Segal AM. Methotrexate in the treatment of arthritis and connective tissue diseases. Cleve Clin J Med 1987;54:327.

68. Hoffman GS, Cid MC, Hellman DB, et al. A multicenter, randomized, double-blind, placebo-controlled trial of adjuvant methotrexate treatment for giant cell arteritis. Arthritis Rheum 2002;46:1309.

69. Cantini F, Niccoli L, Salvarani C, et al. Treatment of longstanding active giant cell arteritis with infliximab: report of four cases. Arthritis Rheum 2001;44:2933.

70. Paulley JW, Hughes JP. Giant-cell arteritis or arteritis of the aged. BMJ 1960;2:1552.

15

Thyroid-Associated Orbitopathy

OVERVIEW

Thyroid-associated ophthalmopathy (TAO) is a common problem in neuro-ophthalmology practices; the presenting complaints are most often diplopia, proptosis, or loss of vision. Nonspecific ocular irritation is frequent, and cosmetic concerns are almost universal, even if not voiced. The "NO SPECS" classification of TAO permeates the medical literature (Table 15-1). Although useful as a mnemonic, this classification is misleading because it falsely implies progression from one stage to the other. It is much more common to have combinations of the various stages, with others excluded, or isolated presentations, such as only stage 3 or stage 4. (See Bartley and Gorman [1] and Liu and Feldon [2] for a detailed discussion of diagnostic criteria.)

TAO affects women three to eight times as often as men. The mean age of onset is 40 years with a wide range (8-80 years). Ocular motility impairment, soft tissue signs, and optic neuropathy are more severe and more common in individuals older than 50 years of age and in men [3]. When eye involvement occurs in childhood Graves' disease, the symptoms and signs tend to be mild [4]. Cigarette smoking is a risk factor for the development of TAO, especially in women, but the mechanism is unknown. Treatment of Graves' disease with radioactive iodine can worsen TAO in certain cases, especially in smokers and in those with significant TAO at the time of treatment [5,6]. The use of prednisone in tapering doses may prevent Iodine-131–induced TAO worsening [5-7].

The ophthalmic manifestations are related to an autoimmune inflammatory process involving antibodies to thyroid-stimulating hormone receptor and other autoantigens present in the orbit, probably

Table 15-1   "NO SPECS" Classification of Thyroid-Associated Ophthalmopathy

Class	Signs
0	No signs or symptoms
1	Only signs (e.g., lid retraction, lid lag, stare)
2	Soft tissue involvement with signs and symptoms (e.g., lid edema, conjunctival chemosis, hyperemia over horizontal rectus muscle insertions, superior limbic keratoconjunctivitis)
3	Proptosis
4	Extraocular muscle involvement
5	Corneal involvement (secondary to exposure)
6	Sight loss (caused by optic nerve compression at orbital apex)

on orbital fibroblasts. The inflammatory response appears to involve both cellular and humoral arms of the immune system, ultimately leading to increased glycosaminoglycan production, increased orbital volume, and fibrosis of the eye muscles [8-10]. In approximately 80% of cases, involvement of both the thyroid gland and orbit occurs within 18 months, but the clinical appearance of the two can be separated by as much as 20 years [9-11].

The natural history of TAO has two stages: active and inactive. The active phase lasts from 8 months to 3 years and is the period in which acute and chronic inflammation is present in the lids, conjunctiva, and orbit. In the inactive phase, the eyes are white, but proptosis, diplopia from extraocular muscle fibrosis, and lid abnormalities can persist. Up to 60% of untreated patients have some spontaneous improvement [12], but improvement is inversely related to the severity of signs and symptoms in my (RT) experience. Recurrent TAO develops in approximately 5% of cases and is often triggered by periods of dysthyroidism [9]. For reasons that are not clear, approximately 15% of patients with eye findings of TAO have no other clinical findings or laboratory abnormalities of dysthyroidism. In the older literature, this presentation was often called "euthyroid thyroid eye disease."

HISTORY AND EXAMINATION

A personal and family history with special attention to previous problems such as hyperthyroidism, goiter, diabetes mellitus, ocular myasthenia, and other autoimmune disorders can be useful. The previous use of thyroid supplements or treatment with radioactive iodine should be inquired about specifically. The patient should be questioned about the existence of cold or heat intolerance, nervousness, weight change, atrial fibrillation, and osteoporosis [13].

Supplemental office tests include exophthalmometry, measurements of lid position, forced duction testing, assessment of color vision, quantification of phorias and tropias, Schirmer's test for low tear production, observation of Bell's phenomenon, measurement of intraocular pressure in up-gaze, external photographs, and contrast sensitivity testing.

INVESTIGATIONS
Thyroid Function Tests

Screening tests for thyroid function include free serum thyroxine (T_4) and thyroid-stimulating hormone (TSH; thyrotropin) levels [5,14]. Measurement of free serum triiodothyronine (T_3), thyrotropin receptor antibodies (more commonly, thyroid-stimulating immunoglobulin [TSI]) and antimicrosomal antibodies may be useful [5,15].

Computed Tomography

High-resolution computed tomography (CT) of the orbit is the single most valuable imaging modality for the evaluation of TAO and for excluding other orbital diseases (Box 15-1). CT also provides a good demonstration of bony anatomy of the orbit, which is needed if orbital decompression is planned.

Orbital Ultrasound (Echography), A- and B-Mode

Eye muscle size and reflectivity can be measured with orbital ultrasound (echography), which, when properly used, is very helpful for the evaluation of TAO [16-18].

Magnetic Resonance Imaging

Although magnetic resonance imaging (MRI) is used often in orbital imaging, it has not supplanted CT in the routine evaluation of TAO. However, with the correct pulse sequences to suppress signal from fat, MRI shows soft tissue detail better than CT and is usually more useful in detecting optic nerve compression causing dysthyroid optic neuropathy (DON) [19,20]. MRI may also be useful in detecting disease activity based on T2 signal intensity [21], near-resonance saturation pulse imaging [22], or post-contrast enhancement [23].

DIFFERENTIAL DIAGNOSIS OF THYROID-ASSOCIATED OPHTHALMOPATHY

The differential diagnosis of TAO is described in Box 15-1.

TREATMENT

The goals of treatment for TAO include relief of ocular discomfort, protection of the corneas, elimination of diplopia, and protection or restoration of visual function. Treatment depends not only on the presenting signs and symptoms but also on whether the disease is in the active or inactive phase. Because eye signs and symptoms are attenuated

---

Box 15-1   Differential Diagnosis of Thyroid-Associated Ophthalmopathy

Ocular myasthenia in 10-15%
Orbital tumors
   Primary
      Hemangioma, meningioma, glioma, lymphoma
   Metastatic
      Breast, lung, colon, prostate
Orbital inflammations
   Orbital pseudotumor
   Orbital myositis
   Wegener's granulomatosis
Orbital infections
   Cellulitis
   Trichinosis
   Arteriovenous fistulas
   Low flow dural shunt syndrome

by euthyroidism, every effort should be made to normalize thyroid function as soon as possible [24].

Patients in the active stage of the disease respond best to immunologic suppression and orbital irradiation. In this regard, prednisone and orbital irradiation have been found about equally effective in patients with moderately severe, previously untreated TAO [25]. In selected cases, steroids are administered intravenously or orally [26,27].

Some believe that combining radiation with oral prednisone is better than either agent alone. The risk of radiation retinopathy is small but real [28,29]. Because of the similarity between diabetic retinopathy and radiation retinopathy, diabetes mellitus is considered a contraindication to orbital irradiation for TAO [30,31].

The usefulness of orbital irradiation for TAO has recently been questioned by Gorman and colleagues [32]. However, their study is flawed by broad inclusion criteria, varied timing of irradiation with respect to the onset of signs and symptoms of TAO, and lack of control for the previous use of steroids. My experience suggests that irradiation or steroids can be useful for selected patients in the active inflammatory stages of TAO. However, radiation therapy alone does not seem to resolve diplopia from TAO [33].

Bromocriptine, a dopaminergic drug, has been tested in the treatment of acute TAO [34]. It is recommended only for patients with combined elevation of TSH and prolactin levels. At least 6 weeks of treatment are needed before clinical effects are seen.

With the exception of orbital decompression for compressive optic neuropathy or for severe proptosis, most surgical techniques for TAO require a stability of findings for at least 6 months [35]. Exceptions can be made if ocular motility is changing rapidly for the worse [36]. If orbital decompression, extraocular muscle surgery, and lid surgery are all indicated, they should be performed in that order because strabismus following orbital decompression is very common [36].

External Signs and Symptoms

Periorbital edema is treated by elevation of the head at night, either by multiple pillows or by elevating the head of the bed on blocks. Diuretics have been used to reduce fluid accumulation, but their effects are transitory. Ocular irritation resulting from lagophthalmos, corneal irritation, and conjunctival involvement are treated using tear substitutes during the day and lubricant ointments at night. If nocturnal lagophthalmos is severe, taping the lids shut or using moisture shields at night has been recommended. Tarsorrhaphy or other lid surgery may be necessary. Tinted lenses are suggested for patients with photophobia.

Eyelid Retraction

Pathologic lid retraction, involving the upper or lower lids or both, occurs in approximately 50% of patients with TAO and poses problems for cosmesis, blinking, and anterior segment exposure. Concomitant proptosis is an aggravating factor. The mechanisms for lid retraction in

TAO include: (1) direct inflammatory involvement of the levator muscle [37]; (2) hyperactivity of the sympathetic nervous system in hyperthyroidism with activation of Mueller's muscle; and (3) secondary overaction of the levator and superior rectus complex in response to involvement and restriction of the inferior rectus muscle [38].

A number of surgical procedures for lid retraction in TAO exist. These include anterior and posterior approaches for levator aponeurosis disinsertion or recession, and the use of spacer material interposed between the levator aponeurosis and the tarsus or the lower lid retractors and tarsus. Extirpation of Mueller's muscle or recession of the inferior rectus to lessen secondary deviation of the levator also may be appropriate [35,39]. Injection of botulinum toxin into the conjunctiva at the superior margin of the tarsal plate has been recommended for TAO-associated lid retraction [40].

Extraocular Muscle Involvement

The frequency of symptomatic rectus muscle involvement in TAO is: inferior rectus; medial rectus; superior rectus; and, very rarely, lateral rectus. Inferior rectus involvement leads to hypotropia and pseudo double-elevator palsy (Box 15-2).

Medial rectus involvement presents as esotropia and may mimic a chronic sixth cranial nerve palsy or Duane's retraction syndrome. Superior rectus dysfunction in TAO is rare (about 10%) and results in hypertropia. As noted previously, involvement of this muscle may be part of the explanation for the pathologic lid retraction of TAO. Lateral rectus fibrosis leads to exotropia, and may be confused with a pupil-sparing third cranial nerve palsy. Lymphoma, focal metastasis, and myositis should be considered, especially when the lateral rectus is involved. Early involvement of any of the recti may present with rather full versional eye movements and unimpressive forced ductions. With any atypical presentation of TAO ocular myasthenia must be kept in mind, especially if exotropia is present.

The diplopia associated with eye muscle involvement in TAO is often managed with prisms, either pressed on (Fresnel) or ground into lenses (see Chapter 3). The choice will depend on the magnitude of the deviation and its stability. Surgical recession of the involved muscle, with or without adjustable suture technique, is usually reserved for cases that have a stable deviation for at least 6 months. Exceptions may be made when the deviation is rapidly progressing for the worse because of muscle fibrosis [36]. Prendiville and co-workers have proposed an approach to vertical strabismus surgery that takes into account restricted ductions as

---

Box 15-2   Other Ocular Motility Signs of Thyroid-Associated Ophthalmopathy

Pseudo double-elevator palsy
Convergence insufficiency
Acquired Brown's syndrome

well as the degree of ocular misalignment [41]. Botulinum toxin injected into the extraocular muscles, with or without eye muscle recession, has been used but is not routine in TAO because of its limited effect.

Optic Nerve Compression

Dysthyroid optic neuropathy (DON) is caused by compression of the optic nerve at the orbital apex by swollen eye muscles, occurring in 5-8% of those with TAO. Signs and symptoms are typical for any compressive optic neuropathy: (1) slow to insidious onset; (2) lack of significant pain; (3) visual field defects; (4) relative afferent pupillary defect if the process is asymmetric or unilateral; (5) color vision abnormalities; and (6) abnormal contrast sensitivity. Impairment of color vision is often disproportionately more severe than is loss of visual acuity. Congestive signs are usually moderate in patients with DON [42]. Optic disc edema is present in approximately 50% of cases.

Glucocorticoids, orbital irradiation, and orbital decompression have all been used in the treatment of DON. Relapses are reported after all three modes of therapy but are far less frequent and severe after orbital decompression [43-46]. Irrespective of the initial mode of therapy, clinical improvement should occur within 1 month of beginning any treatment [43]. Similarly, relapses most often occur during the first month after treatment cessation [43].

REFERENCES
1. Bartley GB, Gorman CA. Diagnostic criteria for Graves' ophthalmopathy. Am J Ophthalmol 1995;119:792.
2. Liu D, Feldon S. Thyroid ophthalmopathy. Ophthalmol Clin North Am 1992;5:597.
3. Kendler DL, Lippa J, Rootman J. The initial clinical characteristics of Graves' orbitopathy vary with age and sex. Arch Ophthalmol 1993;111:197.
4. Chan W, Wong GW, Fan DS, et al. Ophthalmopathy in childhood Graves' disease. Br J Ophthalmol 2002;86:740.
5. Weetman AP. Graves' disease. N Engl J Med 2000;343:1236.
6. Bonnema SJ, Bartalena L, Toft AD, Hegedus L. Controversies in radioiodine therapy: relation to ophthalmopathy, the possible radioprotective effect of antithyroid drugs, and use in large goitres. Eur J Endocrinol 2002;147:1.
7. Rasmussen AK, Nygaard B, Feldt-Rasmussen U. (131)-I and thyroid-associated ophthalmopathy. Eur J Endocrinol 2000;143:155.
8. Hufnagel TJ, Hickey WF, Cobbs WH, et al. Immunohistochemical and ultrastructural studies on the exenterated orbital tissues of a patient with Graves' disease. Ophthalmology 1984;91:1411.
9. Kazim M, Goldberg RA, Smith TJ. Insights into the pathogenesis of thyroid associated orbitopathy. Arch Ophthalmol 2002;120:380.
10. Hatton MP, Rubin PA. The pathophysiology of thyroid-associated ophthalmopathy. Ophthamol Clin North Am 2002;15:113.
11. Kalmann R, Mourits MP. Late recurrence of unilateral Graves' orbitopathy on the contralateral side. Am J Ophthalmol 2002;133:727.
12. Perros P, Crombie AL, Kendaltaylor P. Natural history of thyroid associated ophthal-mopathy. Clin Endocrinol (Oxf) 1995;42:45.
13. Smith SA. Commonly asked questions about thyroid function. Mayo Clin Proc 1995;70:573.

14. Toft AD. Subclinical hyperthyroidism. N Engl J Med 2001;345:512.
15. Saravanan P, Dayan CM. Thyroid autoantibodies. Endocrin Metabol Clin 2001;30:315.
16. Carter JA, Utiger RD. The ophthalmopathy of Graves' disease. Annu Rev Med 1992;43:487.
17. Delint PJ, Mourits MP, Kerlen CH, et al. B-scan ultrasonography in Graves' orbitopathy. Doc Ophthalmol 1993;85:1.
18. Prummel MF, Suttorp-Schulten MSA, Wiersinga WM, et al. A new ultra-sonographic method to detect disease activity and predict response to immunosuppressive treatment in Graves' ophthalmopathy. Ophthalmology 1993a;100:556.
19. Laitt RD, Hoh B, Wakeley C, et al. The value of the short tau inversion recovery sequence in magnetic resonance imaging of thyroid eye disease. Br J Radiol 1994;67:244.
20. Nianiaris N, Hurwitz JJ, Chen JC, et al. Correlation between computed tomography and magnetic resonance imaging in Graves' orbitopathy. Can J Ophthalmol 1994;29:9.
21. Yokoyama N, Nagataki S, Uetani M, et al. Role of magnetic resonance imaging in the assessment of disease activity in thyroid-associated ophthalmopathy. Thyroid 2002;12:223.
22. Ulmer JL, Logani SC, Mark LP, et al. Near-resonance saturation pulse imaging of the extraocular muscles in thyroid-related ophthalmopathy. Am J Neuroradiol 1998;19:943.
23. Ott M, Breiter N, Albrecht CF et al. Can contrast enhanced MRI predict the response of Graves' ophthalmopathy to orbital radiotherapy? Br J Radiol 2002;75:514.
24. Wiersinga WM, Prummel MF. An evidence-based approach to the treatment of Graves' ophthalmopathy. Endocrin Metab Clin 2000;29:297.
25. Prummel MF, Mourits MP, Blank L, et al. Randomized double-blind trial of prednisone versus radiotherapy in Graves' ophthalmopathy. Lancet 1993b;342:949.
26. Marcocci C. Comparison of the effectiveness and tolerability of intravenous or oral glucocorticoids associated with orbital radiotherapy in the management of severe Graves' ophthalmopathy: results of a prospective, single-blind, randomized study. J Clin Endocrinol Metab 2001;86:3562.
27. Kauppinen-Makelin R, Karma A, Leinonen E, et al. High dose intravenous methylprednisolone pulse therapy versus oral prednisone for thyroid-associated ophthalmopathy. Acta Ophthalmol Scand 2002;80:316.
28. Miller ML, Goldberg SH, Bullock JD. Radiation retinopathy after standard radiotherapy for thyroid-related ophthalmopathy. Am J Ophthalmol 1991;112:600.
29. Noble KG. Central retinal artery occlusion: the presenting sign in radiation retinopathy. Arch Ophthalmol 1994;112:1409.
30. Wiersinga W, Prummel MF. Retrobulbar radiation in Graves' ophthalmopathy. J Clin Endocrinol Metab 1995;80:345.
31. Bartalena L, Maecocci C, Tanda ML, et al. Orbital radiotherapy for Graves' ophthalmopathy. Thyroid 2002;12:245.
32. Gorman CA, Garrity JA, Fatourechi V, et al. The aftermath of orbital radiotherapy for Graves' ophthalmopathy. Ophthalmology 2002;109:2100.
33. Ferris JD, Dawson EL, Plowman N, et al. Radiotherapy in thyroid eye disease: the effect on the field of binocular single vision. J AAPOS 2002;6:71.
34. Lopatynsky MO, Krohel GB. Bromocriptine therapy for thyroid ophthalmopathy. Am J Ophthalmol 1989;107:680.
35. Garrity JA. The surgical management of Graves' ophthalmopathy. Curr Opin Ophthalmol 1994;5:39.
36. Coats DK, Paysse EA, Plager DA, Wallace DK. Early strabismus surgery for thyroid ophthalmopathy. Ophthalmology 1999;106:324.

37. Onishi T, Nogushi S, Murakami N, et al. Levator palpebrae superioris muscle: MR evaluation of enlargement as a cause of upper eyelid retraction in Graves' disease. Radiology 1993;188:115.
38. Hamed LM, Lessner AM. Fixation duress in the pathogenesis of upper eyelid retraction in thyroid orbitopathy. Ophthalmology 1994;101:1608.
39. Maus M, Stefanyszyn MA. Management and surgical review of Graves' ophthalmopathy. Curr Opin Ophthalmol 1992;3:649.
40. Uddin JM, Davies PD. Treatment of upper eyelid retraction associated with thyroid eye disease with subconjunctival botulinum toxin injection. Ophthalmology 2002;109:1183.
41. Prendiville P, Chopra M, Gauderman WJ, Feldon SE. The role of restricted motility in determining outcomes for vertical strabismus surgery in Graves' ophthalmopathy. Ophthalmology 2000;107:545.
42. Trobe JD, Glaser JS, Laflamme P. Dysthyroid optic neuropathy: clinical profile and rationale for management. Arch Ophthalmol 1978;96:1199.
43. Panzo GJ, Tomsak RL. A retrospective review of 26 cases of dysthyroid optic neuropathy. Am J Ophthalmol 1983;96:190.
44. Carter KD, Frueh BR, Hessburg TP, et al. Long-term efficacy of orbital decompression for compressive optic neuropathy of Graves' eye disease. Ophthalmology 1991;98:1435.
45. Fatourechi V, Bergstralh EJ, Garrity JA, et al. Predictors of response to transantral orbital decompression in severe Graves' ophthalmopathy. Mayo Clin Proc 1994;69:841.
46. Feldon SE. Management of Graves' ophthalmopathy with optic nerve involvement. Mayo Clin Proc 1993;68:616.

16

Transient Monocular Blindness

OVERVIEW
Transient monocular blindness (TMB) has a number of etiologies. A useful classification divides TMB into four types according to cause [1]. I (RT) have modified and expanded this classification in Box 16-1 [2-11].

Remember that patients with transient homonymous hemianopias may think that only one eye is involved. In this case they are attributing the vision loss to the larger affected temporal hemifield.

CLINICAL FEATURES
Transient Monocular Blindness from Emboli
These attacks are typically sudden and painless in onset, last 5-15 minutes, and are often accompanied by altitudinal loss of vision described as a "shade" or "curtain" being pulled in front of the eye [1,12-17]. Attacks of TMB from emboli cause photopsias only rarely [17]. According to

---

Box 16-1   Types of Transient Monocular Blindness
TMB from emboli (amaurosis fugax)[a]
Carotid arteries
Aortic arch
Heart valves
Patent foramen ovale
Atheromatous embolism following abdominal surgery, arteriography, or anticoagulation[b]
TMB from retinal or optic nerve hypoperfusion
High-grade carotid stenosis or occlusion (ocular ischemic syndrome)
Steal syndromes
Partial retinal vein occlusion
Optic disc edema
Giant cell arteritis
Hyperviscosity/hypercoagulability syndromes
TMB from retinal vasospasm
Retinal migraine
Retinal vasospasm without migraine headache
Retinal vasospasm in atherosclerotics
TMB from other causes (see Box 16-2)

TMB = transient monocular blindness.
[a]Some purists use "amaurosis fugax" to refer only to TMB of embolic etiology. For an historic overview of this term, see Hankey GJ, Warlow CP. Transient Ischemic Attacks of the Brain and Eye. Major Problems in Neurology (Vol 27). Philadelphia: Saunders, 1994, and Fisher CM. "Transient monocular blindness" versus "amaurosis fugax." Neurology 1989;39:1622.
[b]JW Online. A mimic of vasculitis (atheromatous embolization). Cleve Clin J Med 1992;59:96.

Hankey and Warlow [13], 75-80% of embolic TMB cases have an arterial cause, approximately 20% have a cardiac cause, and less than 5% are due to thromboembolism from hematologic abnormalities.

Three classic types of emboli are described: cholesterol (Hollenhorst's plaques); calcific; and fibrin-platelet (Figure 16-1). Cholesterol emboli are golden in color and often lodge at retinal arterial bifurcations (Figure 16-2) and are shaped much like a tile or shingle. Thus, when examining a patient with TMB, it is useful to gently press on the lower eyelid during ophthalmoscopy because this can sometimes cause a hidden embolus to change its orientation and thus become visible.* Calcific emboli look white or chalky and are rectangular or round; these classically come from the heart but can arise from atherosclerotic large arteries [18]. Platelet-fibrin emboli are yellow-white and tend to fill a portion of the arterial lumen. On occasion these emboli migrate through the retinal circulation [19]. In some patients with previous retinal embolization, damage to the vessel wall occurs, leaving a whitish segment that can be mistaken for a recent embolus.

The presence of asymptomatic retinal emboli as an independent risk factor is associated with an approximate tenfold higher risk of stroke and a 50% increase in the chance of nonfatal myocardial infarction or vascular death within 3 years. Interestingly, retinal infarction was no more common in these patients than in the control group [20-22]. For reasons that are unclear, patients with TMB and carotid artery stenosis

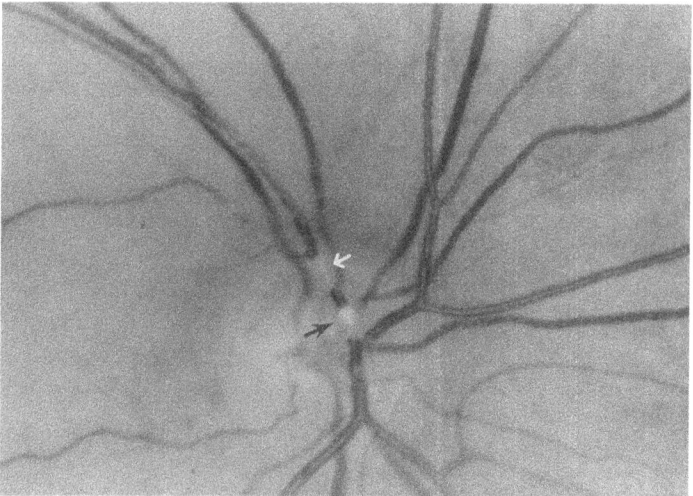

Fig 16-1   Calcific embolus *(black arrow)* and platelet fibrin plug *(white arrow)* in a patient with a superior temporal branch artery occlusion in the left eye. Note segmentation of arterial blood column distal to embolic obstruction.

*Personal communication from E.W.D. Norton, 1979.

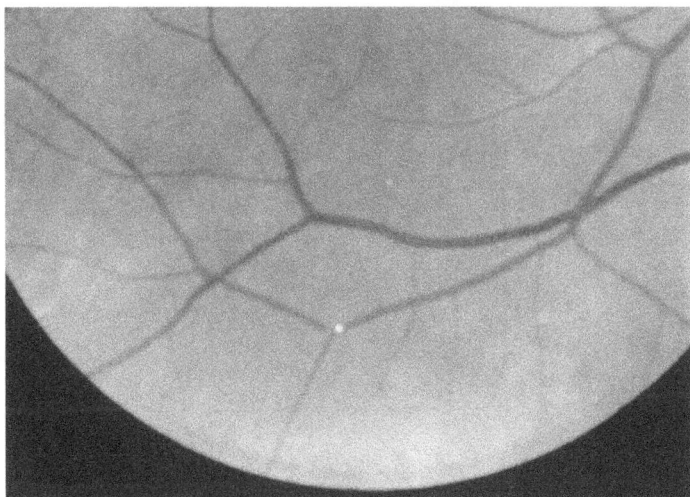

Fig 16-2 Cholesterol embolus (Hollenhorst's plaque) lodged at a bifurcation of the inferotemporal branch artery of the right eye.

have a better prognosis for stroke than those with hemispheric transient ischemic attacks (TIAs) [13,14]. Benavente and colleagues found that the 3-year risk of ipsilateral stroke in medically treated patients who presented with TMB was about half that of those who presented with hemispheric TIAs [14].

Transient Monocular Blindness from Ocular Hypoperfusion

The classic example of this disorder is ocular ischemic syndrome (OIS), in which high-grade carotid stenosis or occlusion leads to chronic ocular ischemia. The symptoms include aching periocular pain; signs of anterior segment ischemia, including ocular hypotension and aqueous humor flare; and signs of retinal ischemia, including midperipheral retinal hemorrhages, posterior pole nerve fiber layer infarcts, and venous dilation (Figure 16-3).

Iris and posterior segment neovascularization can occur. Transient unilateral vision loss in bright light (hemeralopia) is the symptom of relevance to OIS [23]. This occurs presumably because of metabolic impairment of photopigment regeneration caused by hypoxia. This symptom can be thought of as a pathologic variant of the macular photostress phenomenon. Vasospasm may also play a role [24].

A postural form of TMB has been described in patients with giant cell arteritis and extremely tenuous optic disc perfusion [25].

Transient vision obscurations are usually seen in patients with optic disc edema from increased intracranial pressure (papilledema). The vision disturbance may be unilateral or bilateral, lasts seconds, and is often

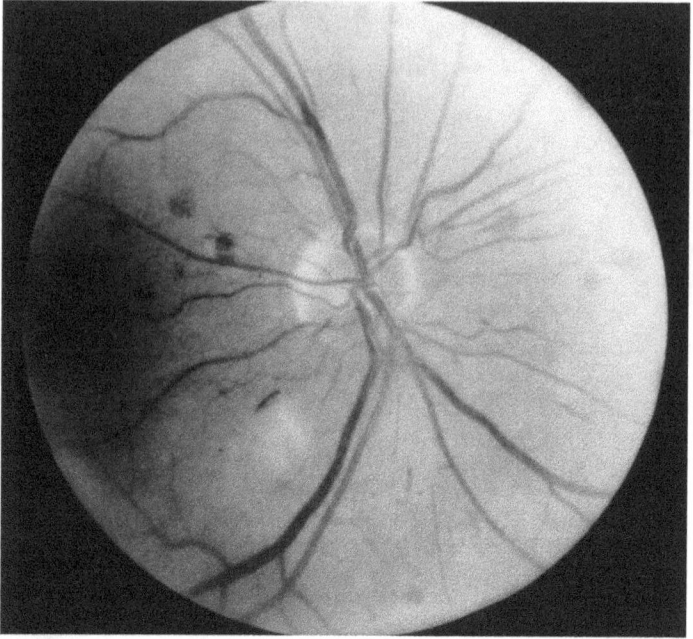

Fig 16-3   Ocular ischemic syndrome. Posterior pole of right eye showing scattered flame-shaped and blot hemorrhages and occasional nerve fiber layer infarcts.

brought on by postural change or straining. The transient conduction block in the optic nerve that gives rise to this symptom is probably caused by axoplasmic flow stasis and transient disc ischemia.

Transient Monocular Blindness from Retinal Vasospasm

TMB can be a consequence of retinal vasospasm [26] and is sometimes called retinal migraine.* Patients with this condition tend to be younger and commonly do not have risk factors for embolic or atherosclerotic disease; although increased platelet aggregability may play a role [28,29]. Retinal vasospasm may be longer lasting than other forms of TMB and may be accompanied by positive visual phenomenon (photopsias). The vision loss often begins as concentric constriction of the visual field indicative of generalized ocular hypoperfusion [13]. Postural change or exercise may bring on vision loss, and a mild aching sensation around the eye is often mentioned by those affected [30].

Vasospastic amaurosis fugax has been described in adults with atherosclerosis and other risk factors [31,32]. According to one estimate, vasospasm may be responsible for up to 10% of cerebral TIAs [33].

---

*The International Headache Society Classification requires that headache be a part of a retinal migraine attack (IHS 1.4) [27].

Abnormalities in the synthesis and release of nitric oxide are probably responsible for many of these phenomena [34].

Transient Monocular Blindness from Other Causes

Subacute attacks of angle-closure glaucoma should also be considered in the differential diagnosis of temporary monocular vision loss, especially if the patient complains of halos around lights [2]. This symptom results from corneal edema related to rapid elevations of intraocular pressure and may not be associated with eye pain or redness.

Temporary loss of vision with elevation of body temperature (Uhthoff's symptom) is most often seen in patients with optic neuritis from demyelinating disease [3] but may accompany other disorders such as Leber's hereditary optic neuropathy, Friedreich's ataxia, and suprasellar tumors [17].

Recurrent remitting vision loss has also been described with orbital tumors (gaze-evoked amaurosis) and intracranial masses, including sphenoid sinus mucocele, craniopharyngioma, pituitary adenoma, and oligodendroglioma [4-9].

In patients with vague monocular or alternating visual symptoms, corneal epithelial basement membrane dystrophy needs to be excluded as a cause [10].

Wray [1] notes that some young patients with TMB can have circulating antiphospholipid antibodies sometimes associated with splinter hemorrhages in the fingernail beds. Donders and colleagues found that the prevalence of TMB in those with systemic lupus erythematosus (SLE) was approximately 11 times greater than that in normal subjects, but they could not find an association with the presence of antiphospholipid antibodies and TMB in the SLE group [35].

TMB has been reported in a patient with a partial central retinal vein occlusion and ocular hypertension. Symptoms resolved coincident with decreasing intraocular pressure with use of beta-blocker eye drops [36].

Finally, any patient with vision disturbance may have TMB from nonorganic causes. This diagnosis should be one of exclusion, in any case.

INVESTIGATIONS
Transient Monocular Blindness from Emboli

These patients not only need to be evaluated for carotid and cardiac valvular disease (Box 16-2) but also need a medical evaluation for hypertension, hyperlipidemia, coronary artery disease, and peripheral vascular disease because of the high prevalence of these conditions in patients with TIAs [13]. Echocardiography is also successful in identifying proximal lesions in the proximal aortic arch [37-39].

Transient Monocular Blindness from Ocular Hypoperfusion

The major cause for symptoms in this category is OIS, and the evaluation is described in Table 16-1 [11]. Asymmetric diabetic retinopathy and

Box 16-2   Some Investigations for Embolic Transient Monocular Blindness

History and physical examination including auscultation of carotid vessels and heart
Blood work including lipid, C-reactive protein, and fibrinogen[a] levels
Noninvasive carotid studies
    Doppler or ultrasound
    Phonoangiography
    Magnetic resonance angiography
Conventional intra-arterial arteriography
Other
    Ophthalmodynamometry
    Periorbital Doppler[b]
    Oculoplethysmography
    Color Doppler of ophthalmic artery blood flow
    Echo cardiography (especially transesophageal)

[a]Elevated fibrinogen level is an independent risk factor for stroke. See Tanne D, Benderly M, Goldbourt U, et al. A prospective study of plasma fibrinogen levels and the risk of stroke among participants in the bezafibrate infarction prevention study. Am J Med 2001;111:457.
[b]Repo LP, Suhonen MT, Terasvirta ME, et al. Color Doppler imaging of the ophthalmic artery blood flow spectra of patients who have had a transient ischemic attack. Ophthalmology 1995; 102:1199.

Table 16-1   Transient Monocular Blindness from Other Causes

Cause	Reference
Subacute angle closure glaucoma	2
Uhthoff's symptom in optic neuritis	3
Cystic intracranial tumors	4-9
Orbital neoplasms (gaze-evoked TMB)	6
Recurrent microhyphema	
Corneal epithelial basement membrane dystrophy	10
Associated with antiphospholipid antibodies	
Disc elevation	11
Functional visual disturbances	

partial central retinal vein occlusion (CRVO) are part of the differential diagnosis, and a quick way of sorting these possibilities out is through office estimation of retinal artery pressure (ophthalmodynamometry). In OIS retinal artery pressures are very low. Therefore, it is useful to observe the central retinal artery for pulsations ophthalmoscopically as pressure is applied to the globe. Production of diastolic retinal artery pulsations will require a fair amount of digital pressure in diabetic retinopathy and partial CRVO, but the central retinal artery will collapse with very little pressure in OIS.

Transient Monocular Blindness from Retinal Vasospasm

In most cases TMB from retinal vasospasm is a benign condition, especially in patients younger than 40 years of age. In older patients, it is a diagnosis of exclusion. A history regarding migraine or Raynaud's should be obtained. If the patient is having frequent attacks, or if they can be precipitated by a specific maneuver, consideration should be given to attempting fundus fluorescein angiography during the attack [26].

Transient Monocular Blindness from Other Causes

Antiphospholipid antibodies and lupus anticoagulant can be measured directly or indirectly by ordering the Venereal Disease Research Laboratories (VDRL) test and partial thromboplastin time (PTT). Because of the association with systemic lupus erythematosus an antinuclear antibody test should be ordered as well.

A careful slit-lamp examination is necessary to confirm the ocular causes of TMB listed in Table 16-1.

TREATMENT

Any patient with recurrent TMB, no matter the cause, should be instructed in intermittent digital massage of the globe.*

Transient Monocular Blindness from Emboli

In addition to aspirin, a number of antiplatelet agents have been studied and used for TIAs (11). These include dipyridamole (Persantine), sulfinpyrazone (Anturane), ticlopidine (Ticlid), and other nonsteroidal anti-inflammatory drugs. Antiplatelet therapy results in an approximate 25% reduction in risk of stroke and other cardiovascular events, including vascular death and myocardial infarction. At this time, aspirin is the drug of choice because it is inexpensive and no other antiplatelet treatment has been shown more effective. The recommended dose is between 50 and 1500 mg per day [28], but the most common dose prescribed in the United States is 325 mg with enteric coating [21].

Anticoagulation with heparin is usually reserved for patients with crescendo TIAs and surgical contraindications, but no medical contraindications [13]. Warfarin (Coumadin) is most often selected in patients with TIAs from atrial fibrillation [13].

The topic of carotid endarterectomy (CE) in patients with TIAs can be very controversial. In general, in those patients with high-grade stenosis (70-99%) who are fit surgical candidates, CE is suggested if the operating center has an acceptable complication rate [13]. With regard to TMB as the TIA symptom, CE favorably altered the prognosis only if three or more of the following factors were present: 75 years of age or older; male gender; history of hemispheric TIA or hemispheric stroke; history of intermittent leg claudication; ipsilateral internal carotid stenosis greater than or equal to 80%; and no collateral vessels demonstrated by angiography [4]. It is important to evaluate patients presenting with TMB promptly because if the TMB actually is a TIA, the risk of stroke is greatly elevated during the first 30 days after onset [22].

---

*I recommend alternating 5 seconds of moderately vigorous digital massage through closed eyelids with 10 seconds of rest until vision returns. This treatment will lower intraocular pressure, thereby improving retinal and optic nerve perfusion pressure. It also has the potential to dislodge emboli and move them further peripherally in the retinal circulation.

Box 16-3 Treatments for Causes of Embolic Transient Monocular Blindness

Antiplatelet therapy (e.g., enteric-coated aspirin 325 mg/day)
Anticoagulant therapy
Surgery
   Carotid endarterectomy
   Transluminal angioplasty

For extensive discussion see Hankey GJ, Warlow CP. Transient Ischemic Attacks of the Brain and Eye. Major Problems in Neurology (Vol 27). Philadelphia: Saunders 1994, and Tuhrim S. Management of stroke and transient ischemic attack. Mt Sinai J Med 2002;69:121.

Box 16-4 Treatment of Transient Monocular Blindness from Retinal Vasospasm

Calcium channel blockers
Aspirin
Amitriptyline
Topical beta blockers
Isoproterenol inhalation

Transluminal carotid angioplasty is a promising technique but not fully studied. See Box 16-3 for a summary.

Transient Monocular Blindness from Ocular Hypoperfusion

TMB associated with OIS is generally not treated by carotid endarterectomy. In certain selected cases, extracranial-intracranial bypass surgery can improve ocular hemodynamics and aid resolution of the eye signs of ischemia [40]. Winterkorn and Beckman [24] successfully treated one case of OIS with verapamil, a calcium channel blocker.

Ocular complications of OIS, such as neovascular glaucoma, need to be managed by an ophthalmologist.

Transient Monocular Blindness from Retinal Vasospasm

Current evidence suggests that calcium channel blockers such as verapamil (Calan, 120 mg per day) and nifedipine (Procardia, 60 mg per day) are worth trying in patients with TMB unless otherwise contraindicated [31]. Antiplatelet therapy with aspirin also makes sense in these patients. Amitriptyline may have vasorelaxant properties [41]. Timolol eye drops had a salutary effect on one patient's visual migraines [42]. Isoproterenol inhalation aborted migrainous TMB in three patients [43]. See Box 16-4 for a list of treatments for TMB from retinal vasospasm.

REFERENCES

1. Wray SH. Amaurosis fugax. In Tusa RJ, Newman SA (eds), Neuro-Ophthalmological Disorders: Diagnostic Work-up and Management. New York: Marcel Dekker, 1995;3.
2. Ravits J, Seybold ME. Transient monocular visual loss from narrow-angle glaucoma. Arch Neurol 1984;41:991.

3. Selhorst JB, Saul RF. Uhthoff and his symptom. J Neuroophthalmol 1995;15:63.
4. Cogan DG. Blackouts not obviously due to carotid occlusion. Arch Ophthalmol 1961;66:56.
5. Friesen L, Sjostrand J, Norrsell K, et al. Cyclic compression of the intracranial optic nerve: patterns of visual failure and recovery. J Neurol Neurosurg Psychiatry 1976;39:1109.
6. Orcutt JC, Tucker WM, Mills RP, et al. Gaze-evoked amaurosis. Ophthalmology 1987;94:213.
7. McDonald WI. The symptomatology of tumors of the anterior visual pathways. Can J Neurol Sci 1982;8:381.
8. Manor RS, Ben Sira I. Amaurosis fugax at downward gaze. Surv Ophthalmol 1987;31:411.
9. Dirr LY, Troost BT, Elster AD, et al. Amaurosis fugax due to pituitary tumor. J Clin Neuroophthalmol 1991;11:254.
10. Reed JW, Jacoby BG, Weaver RG. Corneal epithelial basement membrane dystrophy: an overlooked cause of painless visual disturbances. Ann Ophthalmol 1992;24:471.
11. Sadun A, Currie JN, Lessell S. Transient visual obscurations with elevated optic discs. Ann Neurol 1984;16:489.
12. Olin JW. A mimic of vasculitis (atheromatous embolization). Cleve Clin J Med 1992;59:96.
13. Hankey GJ, Warlow CP. Transient ischemic attacks of the brain and eye. In Major Problems in Neurology (Vol 27). Philadelphia: Saunders, 1994.
14. Benavente O, Eliasziw M, Streifler JY, et al. Prognosis after transient monocular blindness associated with carotid artery stenosis. N Engl J Med 2001;345:1084.
15. Goodwin JA, Gorelick PB, Helgason CM. Symptoms of amaurosis fugax in atherosclerotic carotid artery disease. Neurology 1987;37:829.
16. Ewing CC. Recurrent monocular blindness. Lancet 1968;1:1035.
17. Donders RC. Clinical features of transient monocular blindness and the likelihood of atherosclerotic lesions of the internal carotid artery. J Neurol Neurosurg Psychiatry 2001;71:247.
18. Winterkorn JMS, Ptachewich Y. Calcific retinal emboli and collateral shunting in a woman with rheumatic heart disease. Arch Ophthalmol 1995;113:1464.
19. Jarrett WH, II, North AW. Dynamic platelet embolization of the retinal arteriole. Arch Ophthalmol 1995;113:531.
20. Bruno A, Jones WL, Austin JK, et al. Vascular outcome in men with asymptomatic retinal cholesterol emboli: a cohort study. Ann Intern Med 1995;122:249.
21. Tuhrim S. Management of stroke and transient ischemic attack. Mt Sinai J Med 2002;69:121.
22. Whisnant JP, Wiebers DO, O'Fallon WM, et al. Effect of time since onset of risk factors on the occurrence of ischemic stroke. Neurology 2002;58:787.
23. Furlan AJ, Whisnant JP, Kearns TP. Unilateral visual loss in bright light. Arch Neurol 1979;36:675.
24. Winterkorn JMS, Beckman RL. Recovery from ocular ischemic syndrome after treatment with verapamil. J Neuroophthalmol 1995;15:209.
25. Wykes WN, Adams GGW, Cullen JF. Temporal arteritis: visual loss associated with posture. Neuroophthalmology 1984;4:107.
26. Kline LB, Kelly CL. Ocular migraine in a patient with cluster headache. Headache 1980;20:253.
27. Headache Classification Committee of the International Headache Society. Classification and diagnostic criteria for headache disorders, cranial neuralgias and facial pain. Cephalgia 1988;8(Suppl 7):1.
28. Johnson ES, Lanes SF, Wentworth CE, et al. A metaregression analysis of the dose-response effect of aspirin on stroke. Arch Int Med 1999;159:1248.

29. Poole CJM, Russell RW, Harrison P, et al. Amaurosis fugax under the age of 40 years. J Neurol Neurosurg Psychiatry 1987;50:81.

30. Tomsak RL, Jergens PB. Benign recurrent transient monocular blindness: a possible variant of acephalgic migraine. Headache 1987;27:66.

31. Winterkorn JMS, Kupersmith MJ, Wirtschafter JD, et al. Brief report: treatment of vasospastic amaurosis fugax with calcium channel blockers. N Engl J Med 1993;329:396.

32. Burger SK, Saul RF, Selhorst JB, et al. Transient monocular blindness caused by vasospasm. N Engl J Med 1991;325:870.

33. Friburg L, Olsen TS. Cerebrovascular instability in a subset of patients with stroke and transient ischemic attack. Arch Neurol 1991;48:1026.

34. Harrison DG. Alterations of vasomotor regulation in atherosclerosis. Cardiovasc Drugs Ther 1995;9:55.

35. Donders RC, Kappelle LJ, Derksen RH, et al. Transient monocular blindness and antiphospholipid antibodies in systemic lupus erythematosus. Neurology 1998;51:535.

36. Loff HJ, Parker K, Tomsak RL. Transient monocular blindness with perfused incomplete retinal vein occlusion. Neuroophthalmology 1994;14:49.

37. Mouradian M, Wijman CA, Tomasian D, et al. Echocardiographic findings of patients with retinal ischemia or embolism. J Neuroimaging 2002;12:219-23.

38. Ernst E. Fibrinogen-an important risk factor for atherothrombotic diseases. Ann Med 1994;26:15.

39. Repo LP, Suhonen MT, Terasvirta ME, et al. Color Doppler imaging of the ophthalmic artery blood flow spectra of patients who have had a transient ischemic attack. Ophthalmology 1995;102:1199.

40. Standefer M, Little JR, Tomsak RL, et al. Improvement in the retinal circulation after superficial temporal to middle cerebral artery bypass. Neurosurgery 1985;16:525.

41. Solomon GD. Pharmacology and use of headache medications. Cleve Clin J Med 1990;57:627.

42. Cotter PB. Scintillating scotomas relieved with topical timolol. Am J Ophthalmol 1987;104:432.

43. Kupersmith MJ, Hass WK, Chase NE. Isoproterenol treatment of visual symptoms in migraine. Stroke 1979;10:299.

17

Traumatic Optic Neuropathy

OVERVIEW AND ETIOLOGY

Trauma to the optic nerve* can result from direct or indirect causes [1-6]. Direct injury is exemplified by stab wounds and gunshot injuries with primary optic nerve damage. Indirect trauma usually occurs with closed head injury to the ipsilateral brow, cheek, or anterior temporal region of the skull (Figure 17-1).

Common causes of injury are motor vehicle accidents, falls, bicycle accidents, and assaults [3,6]. Indirect injuries to the optic nerve cause loss of vision from a variety of mechanisms including avulsion of the nerve, incomplete tears, intradural hemorrhage, subarachnoid hemorrhage, and intraneural contusion with hemorrhage [1,2]. Secondary lesions include edema and swelling of the optic nerves and chiasm, necrosis

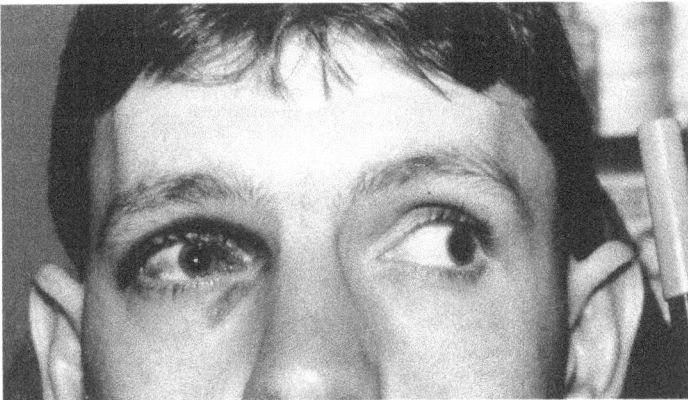

Fig 17-1   Man lost control of compound bow that struck him forcefully in the right periorbital region. Vision was lost immediately (no light perception). On examination, no intraocular abnormalities were found. High-resolution computed tomography of orbits and optic canal was normal. Vision did not improve despite high-dose steroids. Figure shows periorbital ecchymoses and inability to adduct right eye fully because of medical rectus injury. Pupils were pharmacologically dilated.

---

*Hippocrates noted traumatic optic neuropathy: "Dimness of vision occurs in injuries to the brow and in those placed slightly above. It is less noticeable the more recent the wound, but as the scar becomes old so the dimness increases." (From Chadwick J, Mann WN. The Medical Works of Hippocrates. Oxford: Blackwell, 1950;98.)

from systemic circulatory failure or local compression of vessels, and infarction related to thrombosis or arterial spasm [2,4]. It is thought that the intracanalicular portion of the optic nerve is the main site of injury with indirect trauma. Swelling of the nerve in this closed space may be complicated by ischemic changes [6]. Mechanical deformation of the optic canal has been suggested as a cause in some cases [7]. In this regard, Purvin [8] reported the case of a young weight lifter who developed traumatic optic neuropathy after being forced to rest a heavy barbell on his brow after fatiguing during a bench press routine — this injury consisted of a static loading force rather than a blow.

MAIN CLINICAL FEATURES

Vision loss is usually severe and occurs at the time of injury, with the majority of patients left with no light perception [6]. Delayed onset of vision loss over hours to days has been reported [9] (see Case Study). The optic nerve usually appears normal until optic atrophy ensues, but post-traumatic optic disc swelling has been described [10]. See Box 17-1 for a list of the main clinical features of traumatic optic neuropathy (TON).

HISTORY AND EXAMINATION

The presence of a relative afferent pupillary defect (RAPD) is an especially useful sign in comatose patients and in excluding functional vision loss. In one study, the depth of the RAPD correlated with visual prognosis [11]. Patients with 2.1 log units of difference from the unaffected eye had no better than hand movements final vision. Conversely, patients with less than 2.1 log units of difference had an average final acuity of 20/30.

Patients with penetrating injuries or orbital fractures have a poor prognosis for visual improvement [12].

The surgical management of comatose patients with computed tomography (CT) evidence of optic canal or orbital apex damage is a special case with significant ethical overtones, but appears to be effective in some hands [13].

INVESTIGATIONS

High-resolution CT is the neuroimaging test of choice. Optic canal fractures, as determined with CT, are present in approximately 50% of

---

Box 17-1   Main Clinical Features with Traumatic Optic Neuropathy

Sudden, severe visual loss following head trauma
Relative afferent pupillary defect if unilateral or asymmetric
Optic nerve field defects (especially cecocentral scotomas and nerve fiber bundle defects)
Retinal or vitreous abnormalities may be present

cases [6]. The presence of a canal fracture seems to correlate with a worse vision presentation [6,11]. CT can also detect subperiosteal hematomas and intraorbital optic nerve sheath hemorrhages [5].

Magnetic resonance imaging using short inversion time recovery sequences showed high-signal lesions in ten of 11 optic nerves imaged 17 days to 14 years after injury. The case studied 4 days after trauma showed no abnormality [14].

Imaging the optic nerve with ultrasound is useful for detecting optic nerve sheath hemorrhages, especially with the "30-degree test" [5].

DIFFERENTIAL DIAGNOSIS

The two major differential diagnoses are functional vision loss and cortical blindness. Also, vision loss after mild head trauma always raises the possibility of a preexisting mass lesion that was unnoticed before the injury.

TREATMENT

Spontaneous vision improvement occurs with no treatment in 26-50% of patients with traumatic optic neuropathy [6,15,16]. Improvement usually occurs during the first 3 weeks following injury [9].

In a combined series of 223 patients treated with some combination of surgery and corticosteroids, 57% had improvement [6,17]. Patients younger than 40 years of age may respond to optic canal decompression surgery better than patients who are older than 40 years of age [18]. However, as emphasized by Beck and coworkers [19], there are no prospective controlled data to tell if decompression surgery, corticosteroid use, or both actually improve the visual outcome in patients with indirect optic nerve trauma. The most recent nonrandomized report from the International Optic Nerve Trauma Study also suggested no clear benefit of corticosteroids or decompression surgery [20]. However, most experts use one or both of these treatments in selected cases. See, for example, letter from Lee [21].

Possible indications for surgery are shown in Table 17-1. Two similar recommendations for treatment of traumatic optic neuropathy are shown in Box 17-2. These are based, in part, on results of the National Acute Spinal Cord Injury Study II and other experience [22,23]. It is likely that treatment within a few hours of injury is more successful than that started 24 hours or more after the injury [23].

Neuroprotection

The subject of neuroprotection has become very popular in recent years, with the specific aim of thwarting cell death after nervous system injury [24,25]. In regard to TON it is known that apoptosis — "programmed cell death" — is a feature of optic nerve injury in experimental settings and occurs days after the initial trauma [26]. The apoptotic effect may spread to ganglion cells of optic nerve axons that are not primarily injured [27].

Table 17-1 Possible Indications for Surgery in Optic Nerve Trauma

Findings	Surgical Approaches
Subperiosteal orbital hematoma with optic nerve compression	Subperiosteal decompression
Intraorbital hemorrhage with proptosis and vision loss	Lateral canthotomy, cantholysis, possible orbital decompression
Intraorbital optic nerve sheath hemorrhage	Optic nerve sheath fenestration
Delayed or progressive vision loss following indirect optic nerve trauma	Optic canal decompression
Failure of vision improvement after treatment with high-dose IV steroids	Optic canal decompression
Optic canal fracture by computed tomography	Optic canal exploration and decompression

Sources: Spoor TC, McHenry JG. Traumatic Optic Neuropathies. In Tusa RJ, Newman SA (eds), Neuro-Ophthalmological Disorders: Diagnostic Work-up and Management. New York: Marcel Dekker, 1995;99; and Kline LB, Morawetz RB, Swaid SN. Indirect injury of the optic nerve. Neurosurgery 1984;14:756.

Box 17-2 Two Treatment Protocols for Traumatic Optic Neuropathy

Protocol I[a]
IV loading dose of methylprednisolone (30 mg/kg) at onset of diagnosis.
IV methyprednisolone, 5.4 mg/kg/hr for 48 hrs.
If vision improves, oral prednisone in a tapering dose is given.
If no improvement in vision occurs after 48 hrs of IV steroids, surgical decompression of the optic canal is offered.

Protocol 2[b]
Loading dose of IV methylprednisolone (30 mg/kg) at onset of diagnosis.
IV methylprednisolone, 15 mg/kg q6h.
Ranitidine, 150 mg PO bid, is given to prevent gastrointestinal bleeding.
If vision improves, IV therapy is continued for a total of 72 hrs, with rapid taper.
If vision does not improve within 48 hrs, IV treatment is discontinued and optic nerve surgery is offered.

[a]Steinsaper KD, Goldberg RA. Traumatic optic neuropathy. Surv Ophthalmol 1994;38:487.
[b]Spoor TC, McHenry JG. Traumatic Optic Neuropathies. In Tusa RJ, Newman SA (eds), Neuro-Ophthalmological Disorders: Diagnostic Work-up and Management. New York: Marcel Dekker, 1995;99.

A number of neuroprotective drugs are under study — including brimonidine [28], phenytoin [29], and memantine [24] — but none have been proven effective for TON in man.

CASE STUDY

A 51-year-old woman was hit with a tennis ball in the medial canthal region of the right eye and immediately noted loss of vision in the left eye. The injury resulted in a crushed nasal septum and compound nasal fractures. CT of the optic canals was unremarkable. Visual acuity a few hours later was 20/20 OD and 20/30 OS. She was initially treated with oral prednisone, 80 mg per day, for one dose, followed by 40 mg per day for four doses, with no improvement.

Ten days later, vision in her left eye had deteriorated to 20/80. A 3+ left relative afferent pupillary defect was present. Color vision, as tested with Ishihara plates, was normal in the right eye, but she only identified the test plate with the left eye. Visual fields tested by Goldmann technique showed a cecocentral scotoma in the left eye. Funduscopic examination was unremarkable.

Because of visual deterioration, she was treated with three daily doses of intravenous methylprednisolone (IVMP) (1000 mg in 250 cc of normal saline infused over 1 hour each day). Five days later, vision improved to 20/30 OS. Twenty-five days after intravenous treatment was begun, vision was 20/25 OS. Six months later, vision had normalized at 20/20 OS, she identified all of the Ishihara color plates with the left eye, and Octopus (Interzeag, Switzerland) automated perimetry was normal on the left.

Comment

As discussed previously, up to one third of patients with traumatic optic neuropathy improve spontaneously, and it is possible that this patient would have improved with time. However, she was treated with IVMP because of documented visual deterioration. Based on the foregoing, if improvement did not occur rapidly, she would have been a candidate for optic canal decompression.

REFERENCES

1. Lindenberg R, Walsh FB, Sacks JG. Neuropathology of Vision: An Atlas. Philadelphia: Lea & Febiger, 1973;88.
2. Walsh FB. Pathological-clinical correlations. I. Indirect trauma to the optic nerves and chiasm. Invest Ophthalmol Vis Sci 1966;5:433.
3. Kline LB, Morawetz RB, Swaid SN. Indirect injury of the optic nerve. Neurosurgery 1984;14:756.
4. Hedges TR III, Gragoudas ES. Traumatic anterior ischemic optic neuropathy. Ann Ophthalmol 1981;13 (May):625.
5. Spoor TC, McHenry JG. Traumatic Optic Neuropathies. In Tusa RJ, Newman SA (eds), Neuro-Ophthalmological Disorders: Diagnostic Work-up and Management. New York: Marcel Dekker, 1995;99.
6. Steinsaper KD, Goldberg RA. Traumatic optic neuropathy. Surv Ophthalmol 1994;38:487.
7. Gross CE, DeKock JR, Panje WR, et al. Evidence for orbital deformation that may contribute to monocular blindness following minor frontal head trauma. J Neurosurg 1981;55:963.
8. Purvin V. Evidence of orbital deformation in indirect optic nerve injury. Weight lifter's optic neuropathy. J Clin Neuroophthalmol 1988;8:9.
9. Mahapatra AK, Tandon DA. Traumatic optic neuropathy in children—a prospective study. Pediatr Neurosurg 1993;19:34.
10. Brodsky MC, Wald KJ, Chen S, Weiter JJ. Protracted posttraumatic optic disc swelling. Ophthalmology 1995;102:1628.
11. Alford MA, Nerad JA, Carter KD. Predictive value of the initial quantified relative afferent pupillary defect in 19 consecutive patients with traumatic optic neuropathy. Ophthal Plast Reconstr Surg 2001;17:323.
12. Wang BH, Robertson BC, Girotto JA, et al. Traumatic optic neuropathy: a review of 61 patients. Plast Reconstr Surg 2001;107:1655.
13. Lubben B, Stoll W, Grenzebach U. Optic nerve decompression in the comatose and conscious patients after trauma. Laryngoscope 2001;111:320.
14. Takehara S, Tanaka T, Uemura K, et al. Optic nerve injury demonstrated by MRI with STIR sequences. Neuroradiology 1994;36:512.
15. Seiff SR. High dose corticosteroids for treatment of vision loss due to indirect injury to the optic nerve. Ophthal Surg 1990;21:389.

16. Baker SM, Hurwitz JJ. Management of orbital and ocular adnexal trauma. Ophthalmol Clin North Am 1999;12:435.

17. Girard BC, Bouzas EA, Lama SG, et al. Visual improvement after transethmoid-sphenoid decompression in optic nerve injuries. J Clin Neuroophthalmol 1992;12:142.

18. Levin LA, Joseph MP, Rizzo JF III, et al. Optic canal decompression in indirect optic nerve trauma. Ophthalmology 1994;101:566.

19. Beck R, Joseph M, Seiff S, et al. Personal communication from the International Optic Nerve Trauma Study dated January 9,1996.

20. Levin LA, Beck RW, Joseph MP, et al. The treatment of traumatic optic neuropathy: the International Optic Nerve Trauma Study. Ophthalmology 1999;106:1268.

21. Lee AG. Traumatic optic neuropathy (letter). Ophthalmology 2000;107:814.

22. Bracken MB, Shepard MJ, Hellenbrand KG, et al. A randomized, controlled trial of methyl prednisolone or naloxone in the treatment of acute spinal cord injury. Results of the Second National Spinal Cord Injury Study. N Engl J Med 1990;322:1405.

23. McDonald JW, Sadowsky C. Spinal-cord injury. Lancet 2002;359:417.

24. Miller NR. Optic nerve protection, regeneration, and repair in the 21st century: LVIII Edward Jackson Memorial Lecture. Am J Ophthalmol 2001;132:811.

25. Faden AI. Neuroprotection and traumatic brain injury: theoretical option or realistic proposition? Curr Opin Neurol 2002;15:707.

26. Bien A, Seidenbecher CI, Bockers TM, et al. Apoptotic versus necrotic characteristics of retinal ganglion cell death after partial optic nerve injury. J Neurotrauma 16:153.

27. Levkovitch-Verbin H, Quigley HA, Kerrigan-Baumrind LA, et al. Optic nerve transection in monkeys may result in secondary degeneration of retinal ganglion cells. Invest Ophthalmol Vis Sci 2001;42:975.

28. Wheeler LA, Lai R, Woldemussie E. From the lab to the clinic: activation of alpha-2 agonist pathway is neuroprotective in models of retinal and optic neve injury. Eur J Ophthalmol 1999;9 Suppl 1:S17.

29. Naskar R, Quinto K, Romann I, et al. Phenytoin blocks retinal ganglion cell death after partial optic nerve crush. Exp Eye Res 2002;74:747.

II

ORBITAL DISEASE

18

Orbital Disease Evaluation and Differential Diagnosis

OVERVIEW

Orbital diseases are rare, but the differential diagnosis of orbital disease is extensive. Orbital disease can be categorized into five basic clinical patterns: (1) inflammatory; (2) mass effect (causing displacement of globe); (3) structural (major shifts in bony framework); (4) vascular; and (5) functional (decreased vision, afferent pupillary defect or ophthalmoplegia rather than mass effect) [1]. Although many cases can cross over into several categories, most fit predominantly into one of these patterns. A good way to remember all the components in evaluation of orbital disease are the six Ps of orbital disease.

Proptosis

Proptosis [2] is caused by a mass effect and is by far the most typical presentation of orbital disease. Globe displacement, or resistance to retropulsion of the globe are also characteristic. The globe may be displaced axially when the majority of the lesion is within the muscle cone. The globe also may be nonaxially displaced. This is caused by lesions that are mostly outside the muscle cone. This displacement may be superior, inferior, medial, or inferior lateral. Proptosis may be unilateral or bilateral. It also may be confused by pseudoproptosis. The Hertel exophthalmometer accurately measures and follows any amount of proptosis. Race and gender should be kept in mind. The clinician should be suspicious when Hertel measurements show (1) asymmetry of more than 2 mm, (2) whites with measurements of more than 21 mm, and (3) African Americans with measurements of 23 mm or more. Grave's ophthalmopathy is the most common cause of unilateral or bilateral proptosis (Box 18-1).

Progression

Disease progression is very important because it gives the clinical clues to help formulate a differential diagnosis. Acute processes tend to be inflammatory, although aggressive neoplasms must always be ruled out. The opposite is true for chronic disorders—chronic inflammation can pose a diagnostic dilemma because of its insidious infiltrative and cicatrizing characteristic behavior that mimics chronic neoplasia (Box 18-2).

Box 18-1   Types and Possible Causes of Proptosis

Axial Proptosis
Cavernous hemangioma
Optic nerve tumor
Neurilemoma
Arteriovenous malformations
Metastatic tumors to orbital apex[a]
Rhabdomyosarcoma

Superior Displacement
Maxillary sinus tumors

Inferior Displacement
Thyroid eye disease
Capillary hemangioma
Neurofibroma
Lymphoma
Idiopathic orbital inflammation

Down-and-Out Displacement
Dermoid cyst
Frontal sinus mucocele
Osteoma
Frontal sinus tumors

Down-and-In Displacement
Lacrimal gland tumors
Dermoid cyst

Bilateral Proptosis
Thyroid eye disease
Lymphoma
Carotid-cavernous fistula
Neuroblastoma
Idiopathic orbital inflammation
Cavernous sinus thrombosis
Leukemia

Pseudoproptosis
Orbital asymmetry
Globe asymmetry
Palpebral fissure asymmetry
Rectus muscle laxity
Contralateral enophthalmos:
    Metastatic scirrhous breast carcinoma, fracture
    Sick sinus syndrome

[a]May occur anywhere in the orbit.

Pain

Tenderness and sharp pain is typical with an acute inflammatory process, whereas patients with chronic neoplastic infiltration classically feel deep aching pain. Compression by a mass may be perceived as pressure-like pain (Box 18-3).

Palpation

Examination of the fornices and palpation of the orbital quadrants and eversion of the lids may unveil anterior orbital masses. Size, consistency, vascularity, conjunctival, and dermatologic changes should

---

Box 18-2   Progression and Possible Causes of Orbital Disease

Acute Onset (Days to Weeks)
Idiopathic orbital inflammation
Orbital cellulitis
Rhabdomyosarcoma
Neuroblastoma
Metastatic disease
Leukemia

Chronic Gradual Onset (Months to Years)
Dermoid cyst
Pleomorphic adenoma of lacrimal gland
Optic nerve tumors
Peripheral nerve tumors
Cavernous hemangioma

Intermittent Signs and Symptoms
Orbital varix
Orbital lymphangioma
Mucocele
Idiopathic orbital inflammation

---

be evaluated. The location of a lesion may narrow the differential diagnosis (Box 18-4).

Pulsations and Postural Changes

Signs of arterial lesions, such as carotid cavernous fistula or arteriovenous malformations include pulsations with or without bruits, vascular congestion of the periorbital tissues with increased episcleral and intraocular pressure. Conversely, venous lesions, such as orbital varices, are not pulsatile but respond to postural changes that increase venous

---

Box 18-3   Pain in Orbital Disease

Orbital Diseases Frequently Painful
Idiopathic orbital inflammation
Orbital cellulitis
Orbital hemorrhage
Malignant lacrimal gland tumors
Nasopharyngeal carcinoma
Squamous cell carcinoma with perineural invasion[a]

Orbital Diseases Usually Not Painful
Metastatic disease
Orbital abscess
Arteriovenous malformation

Orbital Diseases Rarely Painful
Thyroid disease
Pleomorphic adenoma of the lacrimal gland
Rhabdomyosarcoma
Basal cell carcinoma
Optic nerve tumors
Peripheral nerve tumors

---

[a]See Miller NR, Newman NJ. Basal and squamous carcinoma of the skin. In Miller NR, Newman NJ, (eds.), Walsh and Hoyt's Clinical Neuro-ophthalmology (Vol. 2), (5th Ed). Williams & Wilkins 1998;2457.

Box 18-4   Palpation Findings in Orbital Disease

Superior Nasal Quadrant
Mucocele
Pyocele
Dermoid cyst
Peripheral nerve tumor
Metastatic tumors
Encephalocele

Superior Temporal Quadrant
Lacrimal gland tumor
Dermoid cyst

Inferior Temporal Quadrant
Lymphoma[a]
Idiopathic orbital inflammation[a]

[a]May occur in any quadrant.

pressure (Valsalva maneuvers) (Orcutt JC. Personal communication). (Box 18-5).

Periorbital Changes

Irritation, swelling, pain, warmth, and eventual loss of function suggest inflammatory diseases of the orbit. Nevertheless, the clinician should recognize that masquerade neoplastic lesions could behave similarly. Pain, sclerosis, infiltration, and ischemia may impair extraocular motility restriction. Examination of the eyelids may reveal an S-shaped eyelid, anterior masses, vascular changes, inflammation, and ptosis (Box 18-6).

EXAMINATION

A careful examination includes a complete neuro-ophthalmologic evaluation. A detailed evaluation of the best corrected visual acuity, including refraction, is performed. Color vision is quantified with an Ishihara or Hardy-Rand-Rittler test for color blindness. If this is not available, a test of subjective appreciation of the color red (red desaturation) is helpful. A careful and detailed evaluation of the pupils to find an afferent defect or anisocoria is performed before eye drops are instilled or tonometry is performed. If pupillary asymmetry is found, the pupils are measured in light and dark conditions. Drop testing may be necessary to confirm the diagnosis of Horner's syndrome (cocaine [Paredrine]) or Adie's pupil (dilute pilocarpine). An afferent pupillary defect is graded from 1 to 4 with 4 being the most marked.

Box 18-5   Causes of Pulsating Proptosis

Neurofibromatosis
Following removal of orbital roof
Encephalocele
Carotid-cavernous fistula
Arteriovenous malformation

Box 18-6   Clinical Significance of Systemic, Orbital, Eyelid, Conjuctiva, and Ocular Signs

Systemic

Black eschar in nose	Mucormycoses
Scalp tenderness	Giant cell arteritis

Orbital

Bulging temporal fossa	Sphenoid wing meningioma
Ocular pulsations	Neurofibromatosis, meningoencephalocele
Ocular bruit	Carotid-cavernous fistula, dural fistula
Enophthalmos	Trauma, sinusitis, scirrhous breast carcinoma

Eyelid

S-shaped lid deformity	Plexiform neurofibroma, lacrimal gland mass
Lid lag — lid retraction	Thyroid-related orbitopathy
Prominent veins of lid with proptosis on Valsalva maneuver	Orbital varix
Ecchymosis	Neuroblastoma, leukemia, lymphangioma

Conjunctiva

Salmon patch	Lymphoma
Injection over rectus insertion	Myositis
Dilated and tortuous episcleral vessels	Carotid-cavernous fistula

Ocular

Opticociliary shunt vessels	Meningioma, glioma
Choroidal folds	Orbital pressure

Ocular movement is carefully assessed to determine whether the diplopia is monocular or binocular. Monocular diplopia resolves when a pinhole is placed over the affected eye. Binocular diplopia occurs only when both eyes are used and prevented with occlusion of either eye. Ocular balance is tested in all fields of gaze with the alternate cover test. Nystagmus, if present, is documented.

The position and function of the eyelids relative to the pupil is measured with the marginal reflex distance and the levator muscle excursion (see Ptosis chapter). Retraction of the upper and lower eyelids is noted and measured. The presence of lid lag or lagophthalmus is documented.

Both palpation and Hertel measurements are used to evaluate proptosis. Palpation determines the resistance, particularly the direction of resistance of the globe to a gentle retrodisplacement. All quadrants of the orbit are palpated to feel the anterior portion of any lesions. The orbital rim is assessed for irregularities, expansions, or defects. A Hertel exophthalmometer documents the position of the globe with reference to the orbital rims. The measurements in millimeters of both protrusion and base are recorded. There is a large variation in normal measurements, but an asymmetry greater than 2 mm or an absolute measurement greater than 20 mm may be abnormal [3].

When the evaluation for proptosis is complete, the anterior portions of the adnexa and globe are inspected with a slit lamp. Intraocular pressure is measured in the straight-ahead position and, at times, in a directional position. In evaluation for dysthyroid ophthalmopathy, intraocular pressure tends to increase in the direction opposite the restricted muscle. Therefore, intraocular pressure may be elevated in up-gaze or lateral gaze depending on whether the inferior rectus or the medial rectus is restricted. The cornea is inspected for exposure and the iris is examined for evidence of lesions associated with orbital disease such as Lisch nodules in neurofibromatosis. The lens is inspected for opacification to gain information about the cause of visual dysfunction along with a fundus evaluation. Finally, auscultation of the orbit with a stethoscope listening for bruits is most important.

OTHER INVESTIGATIONS
Laboratory Evaluation
Particularly in the case of inflammatory disease, orbital disorders are often manifestations of systemic abnormalities. Systemic disorders that commonly affect the orbit, and which can be evaluated with laboratory testing, include: Grave's thyroid disease (triiodothyronine, thyroxine, thyroid-stimulating hormone, antimicrosomal, antithyroid receptor, and antithyroglobulin antibodies), sarcoidosis (angiotensin-converting enzyme, chest radiography, serum lysozyme), Wegener's granulomatosis (antinuclear cytoplasmic antibody), myasthenia gravis (acetylcholine receptor antibodies), and lupus erythematosus (antinuclear antibodies).

Visual Fields
Visual fields may be tested in a number of ways. If resources are limited, visual fields can be tested grossly with fingers, tangent screen, or Amsler's grid. In most cases, however, Goldmann or automated perimetry visual fields is essential to document afferent function.

Ultrasonography
Ultrasonography (A and B scans) is a dynamic study that provides infor-mation about the anterior borders of the lesion in respect to its location, configuration, size, and relation to other orbital structures. Ultrasonic A scans provide information about the internal characteristics of the lesion and can provide information regarding the fluid content of the lesion, and with the addition of a Doppler study, the direction of flow of blood in a particular lesion. Ultrasonography, however, lacks the resolution of computed tomography (CT) and magnetic resonance imaging (MRI) in the deep orbit.

Computed Tomography
Computed tomography is the single most important orbital imaging technique to identify anterior orbital and mid-orbital lesions. It is less expensive and more easily obtained compared with an MRI. CT gives detailed information about the location, size, and shape of the orbital and periorbital lesions. It also helps identify bony involvement and the

relation of the lesion to other vital orbital and periorbital structures. The use of contrast medium helps the examiner to see the internal characteristics of the lesions; the specificity of such an exam, however, is less than that of ultrasonography or MRI. To obtain optimal images, the entire orbit should be scanned in fine resolution cuts of 1.5 mm at 1-mm intervals.

Magnetic Resonance Imaging

MRI provides soft tissue and bone marrow resolutions superior to CT and is particularly useful to evaluate tumors of the cavernous sinus and skull base, including optic nerve tumors that enter the cranial cavity. MRIs can be taken in any plane without repositioning the patient. Because bone is not differentiated from air, MRI is not useful in evaluating orbital fractures or differentiating bone and calcium. MRI is better suited than CT to identify the relationship of the tumor to the optic nerve. MRI with gadolinium characterizes the size and configuration of the tumor and the relation of the tumor to other structures in the orbital apex, optic canal, and retro-orbital area. It is also best for evaluating the lesions of the central nervous system that relate to the orbit. Fat suppression is helpful to differentiate orbital lesions from fat and other vital structures. A standard orbital protocol should include axial T1-weighted images without contrast and axial and coronal T1-weighted images after contrast with fat suppression. Magnetic resonance angiography helps to clarify the details of blood flow. Gadolinium (Gd-DTPA) enhancement is used to visualize venous flow, but is not necessary to evaluate arterial flow. Magnetic resonance angiography is used to evaluate intracranial aneurysms, cavernous sinus processes, and vascular processes of the orbit [4].

Tensilon Test

The Tensilon (edrophonium chloride) test is an important office test. The incidence of myasthenia gravis is higher among patients with thyroid disorders. Any patient with unexplained ptosis or motility dysfunction that varies or is atypical in pattern should undergo Tensilon testing. Another method to uncover myasthenia gravis is the "ice test," in which a rubber glove filled with ice or a cold eye pack is placed over the eyes for 5 minutes after which the eye position is checked for improvement. The patient should be questioned about latex allergy if a rubber glove is used (Daroff, R. Personal communication). A "rest test" may be performed, in which the patient is placed in a quiet room with his or her eyes closed and the eyelid position is checked after 5 to 10 minutes.

Forced Duction

The forced duction test differentiates restrictive from paralytic eye movement disorders. This may be accomplished with a forceps after a cotton swab of 4% xylocaine has been applied to the conjunctiva where the forceps is to be placed. If the patient is uncooperative, a Tono-Pen examination is an alternative to forced ductions. Intraocular pressure is measured in primary position in up-gaze away from the action of the

---

Box 18-7   Differential Diagnosis of Enlargement of Rectus Muscles and Optic Nerves

Enlargement of Rectus Muscles
Grave's disease
Carotid-cavernous fistula
Lymphoid tumors
Myositis
Metastatic carcinoma
Sarcoidosis

Enlargement of Optic Nerve
Congenital malformation and cysts
Glioma
Meningioma
Melanocytoma
Angioma
Optic neuritis
Secondary extension of intraocular tumor
Metastatic carcinoma
Chronic papilledema

---

muscle. An increase in intraocular pressure should parallel the tension generated by the restricted muscle (Box 18-7).

Photography

Photographs are essential to document abnormalities. External photographs depict motility disturbance and ptosis, while fundus photographs show abnormalities in the retina, optic nerve, and choroid.

Corticosteroid Trial

Oral corticosteroid, usually prednisone, is inexpensive and effective in the management of acute congestive dysthyroid orbitopathy by decreasing inflammation. It is useful for idiopathic orbital inflammation when initiated at high doses of 80 to 100 mg per day. Although corticosteroids can temporarily decrease the size of a lymphoid lesion, they are not effective as definitive therapy. In idiopathic orbital inflammation, the burden of proof is a needle biopsy or open biopsy to rule out lymphoid lesions.

Orbital Biopsy

Orbital biopsy is definitive in making an accurate diagnosis of orbital disease. Fine needle aspiration biopsy at those centers with skilled cytopathologists is a very useful tool. On the other hand, open biopsy performed with care and skill may get more than sufficient tissue sampling to run the gamut of tests necessary to finalize the diagnosis.

TREATMENT

In the management of orbital disease, orbital imaging is essential before any intervention. MRI and CT are necessary to evaluate the posterior

Box 18-8   Types of Lesions Causing Orbital Disease
Encapsulated Lesions Cavernous hemangioma Neurilemoma Fibrous histiocytoma Pleomorphic adenoma of lacrimal gland Dermoid cyst Leiomyoma Hemangiopericytoma
Diffuse Lesions Idiopathic orbital inflammation Lymphoid tumors Lymphangioma Histiocytosis and xanthomatous lesions Plexiform neuroma Metastatic carcinoma

orbital processes. MRI and CT can be synergistic in diagnosing difficult cases. High-dose corticosteroids with a slow taper are the best management for orbital inflammation. Corticosteroids are not injected into the retrobulbar orbit. Fine needle aspiration biopsy is most helpful to evaluate anterior infiltrative orbital lesions that may be inflammatory or lymphoid proliferations. If incisional biopsy is needed, the most direct approach is used. At least a gram of tissue should be removed for appropriate testing.

In the management of well circumscribed orbital lesions (Box 18-8), attempted total excision through a lateral orbitotomy is performed. If the lesion is located nasally, a medial conjunctival caruncular approach or external medial canthal incision may be combined with a lateral orbitotomy [5]. Anterior superior orbital lesions may be removed with an eyelid crease incision, which is preferable over a sub-brow incision. An inferior lesion may be removed through a transconjunctival approach or subciliary approach [6]. Removal of encapsulated lesions may be accomplished with a finger dissection or direct exposure and instrument dissection. To complete the removal, a cryoprobe may be used.

Nonencapsulated lesions (Box 18-8) cannot be totally excised with preservation of vision. Most of these lesions require a diagnostic biopsy for diagnosis and therapeutic purposes. In some cases a biopsy can be obtained through an anterior approach, but many patients require a lateral orbitotomy. Frozen sections are important to make sure that the biopsy material is representative.

REFERENCES

1. Goldberg RA. Evaluation and spectrum of orbital disease. In Stewart WB (ed). Surgery of the Eyelids, Orbit and Lacrimal System (Vol. 3). San Francisco: American Academy of Ophthalmology, 1995;2.
2. Orbit, Eyelids and Lacrimal System. Basic and Clinical Science Course, 1999-2000, Section 7. San Francisco: American Academy of Ophthalmology.

3. Kennerdell JS, Cuckerham KP, Maroon JC, et al. Practical Diagnosis and Management of Orbital Disease. Boston: Butterworth-Heinemann, 2001;3.
4. Orbit; Eyelids and Lacrimal System. Basic and Clinical Science Course 1999-2000. San Fransico: American Academy of Ophthalmology, 1999;21.
5. Ellis DS, Stewart WB. Lateral orbitotomy. In Levine MR (ed). Manual of Oculoplastic Surgery, (2nd ed). Boston: Butterworth-Heinemann, 1996;291.
6. Spoor TC. Orbital surgery. In Nesi FA, Lisman RD, Levine MR (eds), Smith's Ophthalmic Plastic and Reconstructive Surgery, (2nd Ed). St. Louis: Mosby, 1998;853.

19

Orbital Fractures

OVERVIEW AND ETIOLOGY

Fractures involving the orbit are common. They may be pure blowout fractures or they may have associated fractures. They are caused either by a hydraulic mechanism transmitted by orbital soft tissue energy to the orbital walls or by direct buckling effects of the bony rim or both [1]. The diplopia that takes place is caused by soft tissue entrapment of either muscle, fat, or connective tissue, as described by Kornneef in 1985 [2]. This tissue entrapment occurs when the intraorbital pressure rises after the blow to the orbit causing dissipation of energy 360 degrees to the line of force, which usually is anteriorly to posteriorly directed. In adults with more mature bones (more brittle and less flexible), the thin orbital floor most commonly buckles or blows out toward the maxillary antrum and breaks into several areas. In children or young adults, however, with softer and more flexible bones, the floor is likely to bend, crack, and form a trap door that springs downward and traps tissue, thereby springing back to its normal position [3]. Some surgeons believe that small orbital fractures are more likely to incarcerate extraocular muscles than large fractures and may lead to an ischemic compartment syndrome, which may produce muscle ischemia, fibrosis, and restricted motility [4]. This application may be more significant in the younger patient where tissue entrapment (fat, connective tissue, and muscle) is incarcerated in the flexible trap door fracture. The potential space around the extraocular muscle is disrupted after orbital fractures, and a high compartment pressure occurs around the inferior rectus muscle and ischemia takes place. Therefore, much earlier surgical intervention, within 24 to 48 hours, must be considered for the patient to have a successful outcome. The types of orbital floor fractures are listed in Box 19-1 [5].

CLINICAL SIGNS AND SYMPTOMS

Signs and symptoms of orbital floor fractures are listed in Box 19-2. Diplopia in up- or down-gaze can be due to entrapment of the inferior rectus muscle or, much less often, the inferior oblique muscles, entrapment of orbital fascia or both, and fat with secondary restriction of muscle function. It can also be due to edema and hemorrhage or a subperiosteal hemorrhage. Marked restriction of vertical eye movement is usually associated with linear cracks or flap-type fractures. Generalized restriction in all directions of gaze or in extremes of vertical gaze is often due to edema and hemorrhage. If the inferior rectus muscle is incarcerated anterior to

Box 19-1   Types of Orbital Floor Fractures

Fracture with minimal displacement and no diplopia or enophthalmos
Larger fracture with tissue herniation without diplopia or significant
    enophthalmos
Linear fracture with tight incarceration of tissue restricting ocular motility with
    diplopia
Blowout fracture with herniation and entrapment of tissue, usually causing
    diplopia
A large defect in the bone without tissue entrapment, with severe enophthalmos
    and cosmetic deformity from displacement of the eye usually accompanied
    by diplopia
Orbital floor fractures accompanied by orbital rim or other orbital fractures

the equator of the eye, the eye is hypotropic in primary position with decreased motility in up- and down-gaze. If the fracture with entrapment is at the equatorial part of the globe, the eye is orthophoric in primary position with decreased motility in up- and down-gaze. If the inferior rectus is trapped posterior to the equator of the eye, the eye is hypertropic in primary position with decreased motility in down-gaze because of paresis to the inferior division of the third cranial nerve entering the proximal one-third of the inferior rectus. This allows the superior rectus to act unopposed against the paretic inferior rectus giving the hypertropia.

Pain in attempted up- and down-gaze indicates that with eye movement the muscle or fascia is entrapped or impinged on by the sharp edges of the fractured bone. Infraorbital nerve hypesthesia results from injury to the infraorbital nerve as it traverses the orbital floor. This may be due to compression, edema of the nerve, or partial or complete tearing of the nerve. The hypesthesia usually improves in weeks to months, and on rare occasions, can be permanent.

Periorbital ecchymosis and edema are indicative of blunt trauma and provide some indication of the severity of the injury. If there is no entrapment, improvement in the motility should parallel resolution of the periorbital edema.

Proptosis may be initially caused by retrobulbar edema or hemorrhage and subsequently improves over days to weeks.

Enophthalmos may be caused by any of four mechanisms [6]. (1) A large fracture of the orbital floor may allow orbital fat and other posterior

Box 19-2   Signs and Symptoms of Orbital Floor Fractures

Diplopia
Pain in vertical gaze
Infraorbital nerve hypesthesia
Eyelid ecchymosis
Proptosis
Enophthalmos
Globe ptosis
Subcutaneous emphysema
Epistaxis
Pupillary dilatation

and inferior orbital tissues to prolapse into the maxillary antrum. (2) Bone fragments in the area of the orbital floor can sag into the maxillary antrum, thereby enlarging total orbital volume. The orbital structures, particularly the orbital fat, may expand into this larger volume, thus removing support behind the eye. (3) The inferior rectus muscle can be caught in the fracture at the time of trauma when the orbital contents are compressed into the posterior orbit. The trapped inferior rectus can then tether the globe in this posterior position. (4) Atrophy of the orbital fat after trauma can contribute further to poor support behind the globe, allowing the eye to sink farther back into the orbit.

Globe ptosis is associated with disruption of Lockwood's ligament. A late presentation may be due to inferior displacement of the ligament by fibrosis and contracture. The diagnosis of globe ptosis is based on a comparison with the opposite side, if that eye is not displaced.

Subcutaneous emphysema indicates a communication between a sinus and the orbit. The displacement of air can occur at the time of injury or from resuscitation efforts. The patient suspected of having an orbital fracture should be advised not to blow the nose because this can also cause orbital emphysema. The subcutaneous emphysema usually absorbs over 5 to 7 days without complications.

Epistaxis usually occurs with mucosal tears. It can also occur with damage to the anterior ethmoidal artery.

Pupillary dilatation may occur from injury to the parasympathetic fibers in the portion of the inferior division of the third nerve that travels to the ciliary ganglion near the inferior oblique muscle.

Ocular injuries can also accompany orbital fractures (Box 19-3).

Medial wall fracture should be suspected whenever there is horizontal diplopia, epistaxis, and significant subcutaneous emphysema in the eyelids and orbit after blunt trauma. Although fracture in the medial wall is relatively common, medial rectus entrapment is uncommon. When entrapment does occur, horizontal motility disturbances are observed. There is limitation of abduction resulting from incarceration of the medial rectus, fascia, or fat, but because of the trauma to the muscle, there can be a paresis evident on adduction. If the medial rectus muscle is trapped anterior to the equator of the eye, the eye is generally esotropic

---

Box 19-3   Ocular Injuries

Corneal abrasion
Hyphema
Iridoplegia
Iritis
Lens dislocation
Secondary glaucoma
Cataracts
Vitreous hemorrhage
Retinal hemorrhage and macular edema
Retinal detachment
Choroidal rupture
Optic nerve Injury
Ruptured globe

in primary position with decreased adduction and markedly limited abduction with globe retraction and fissure narrowing. If the medial rectus muscle is trapped at the equator of the eye, the eye is generally straight in primary position with decreased adduction and abduction and less globe retraction and fissure narrowing on abduction. Finally, if the medial rectus muscle is trapped posterior to the equator of the eye, the eye is generally exotropic in primary position with markedly limited adduction and decreased abduction. There is minimal retraction of the globe or narrowing of the palpebral fissure because of lack of involvement of the distal two thirds of the muscle. An explanation for the exotropia is that with posterior entrapment, the nerve to the medial rectus muscle that enters the muscle posteriorly, is traumatized resulting in a temporary paresis of the medial rectus. The combination of a posterior entrapment and paresis, with noninvolvement of the distal two-thirds of the medial rectus allows the direct antagonist (lateral rectus muscle) to act unopposed, causing an exotropia [7].

EXTRAOCULAR MUSCLE TESTS

Evaluation of the extraocular muscle limitation can be done with prism measurements in the cardinal fields of gaze, a red glass test for diplopia, a forced-duction test, an active forced-generation test, and diplopia fields [8]. With a forced-duction test, anesthetic drops are instilled in the eye and toothed forceps are used to grasp the conjunctiva and Tenon's capsule just inferior to the limbus at the 6 o'clock position of the globe. If the patient is limited in up-gaze and the examiner cannot elevate the globe with a forceps, it is likely that entrapped inferior orbital structures are tethering the globe. There are, however, other causes that limit globe movement, such as a superior subperiosteal hematoma and edema of the orbit. A strongly positive forced-duction test is of some help in distinguishing entrapped inferior orbital tissues from other causes, particularly in association with radiographic evidence of an orbital floor fracture. In an active forced-generation test, the relative strength of the inferior rectus muscle may be evaluated by asking the patient to look down while fixing the eye with a toothed forceps. This test is useful for differentiation of paresis from entrapment.

Diplopia fields are obtained binocularly by having the patient follow a small test object with either a Goldmann perimeter or a tangent screen. When the patient states that the test object appears double, the point is plotted. This procedure is continued until the entire field is plotted, noting the area in which there was single vision and that in which there is double vision. This diplopia field can be repeated to determine if improvement has occurred during the early period of observation.

IMAGING STUDIES

Computed tomography (CT) with coronal views is invaluable in the diagnosis and management of orbital floor fractures. CT scanning very effectively shows the size of the fracture as well as the extent of incarceration of extraocular muscle and soft tissues. Axial cuts are not as helpful in delineating fractures. However, axial views are important in evaluating fractures of the medial orbital wall. When a CT scan is not available, a Waters' view of the skull is the best radiologic means for screening patients suspected of having a blowout fracture of the orbital floor. This view may show fragmentation of the bone of the floor, prolapse of orbital soft tissue into the maxillary antrum, fluid due to blood in the maxillary antrum, and sometimes air in the orbit or eyelids. Unfortunately, soft tissue densities visualized within the maxillary sinus may be a hematoma, fat, or muscle and does not prove muscle entrapment.

Finally, magnetic resonance imaging (MRI) shows soft tissue details particularly well, but does not image cortical bone and, therefore, is not very useful in evaluating orbital fractures.

TREATMENT

The overall indication for surgical intervention for blowout fractures remains controversial. Indications for conservative surgery within 10 to 14 days include: (1) vertical diplopia that doesn't improve within 10 to 14 days; (2) a positive forced-duction test; (3) evidence on CT of soft tissue entrapment; (4) early enophthalmos of 3 mm or more; and (5) floor fracture greater than 50% shown on CT scan.

The 10- to 14-day grace period allows for resolution of the initial periorbital and intraorbital edema and hemorrhage. A short course of systemic steroids may quicken this resolution. Improvement of diplopia may also be due to resolution of soft tissue swelling that allows for reduction of entrapped tissue in larger defects. Additionally, surgery at this time is easier due to better exposure and less risk of bleeding.

Immediate surgery is occasionally necessary, as in the case of globe herniation into the maxillary sinus, and also in cases of trap door fractures most commonly seen in pediatric cases. These cases typically present with incarcerated extraocular muscles or septa that can cause ischemic compartment syndrome, fibrosis, and motility restriction. There is a strong link between nausea, vomiting, and bradycardia and trap door fractures [9]. Surgical intervention within 24 to 48 hours would be required, therefore, in the young patient who has minimal soft tissue clinical signs, marked restriction in vertical gaze and forced-duction test, and CT scan evidence of linear fracture with no bone displacement with or without tissue entrapment into the antrum.

The preferred method of repair for blowout fractures is a transconjunctival approach, which provides good exposure, a minimally visible scar, and a reduced incidence of postoperative lower lid retraction and ectropion. Lateral canthotomy and inferior cantholysis improve exposure. An alternate incision is the infraciliary approach, which also provides good exposure, but can cause a visible lid scar and lower lid retraction or ectropion. The goal of the surgery is to reduce the incarcerated contents while visualizing the posterior limits of the fracture, so no residual entrapped tissue remains. An implant is then placed, such as Medpore, Teflon, or Supramid to cover the defect and prevent reherniation or to provide a nonadherent surface to prevent adhesions from forming between the orbital tissues and the bone.

Medial wall fractures are preferably repaired through a medial canthal skin approach. Other surgeons recommend a transconjunctival or caruncular approach to the medial orbit.

REFERENCES

1. Smith B, Regan WF. Blowout fractures of the orbit: mechanism and correction of internal orbital fracture. Am J Ophthalmol 1957;44:733.
2. Kornneef LP. Current concepts on the management of orbital blowout fractures. Ann Plast Surg 1982;9:185.
3. Jordan DR, Allen LH, White J, et al. Intervention within days for some orbital floor fractures: the white-eyed blowout. Ophthal Plast Reconstr Surg 1998;14(6):379.
4. Smith B, Lisman RD, Simonton J, et al. Volkman's contracture of the extraocular muscles following blowout fracture. Plast Reconstr Surg 1984;74:200.
5. Rathbun JE. Orbital fractures. In Stephenson CM (ed). Ophthalmic Plastic Reconstructive and Orbital Surgery. Boston: Butterworth-Heinemann, 1997;417.
6. Hawes MJ, Dortzbach RK. Blowout fractures of the orbital floor. In Dortzbach RK (ed). Ophthalmic Plastic Surgery: Prevention and Management. New York: Raven Press, 1994;195.
7. Allen V, Levine MR. Medial wall fractures. In Hornblass A (ed). Oculoplastic, Orbital and Reconstructive Surgery (Vol. II). Baltimore: Williams & Wilkins, 1990;1168.
8. Dortzbach RK, Kikkawa DO. Blowout fractures of the orbital floor. In Stewart WB (ed). Surgery of the Eyelid, Orbit and Lacrimal System (Vol. 3). San Francisco: American Academy of Ophthalmology 1995;204.
9. Bansagi ZC, Meyer DR. Internal orbital fractures in the pediatric age group. Ophthalmology 2000;107(5):829.

20

Classification and Examination of the Ptosis Patient

ETIOLOGY AND OVERVIEW

Blepharoptosis or ptosis is an abnormal drooping of the eyelids. Beard published the first comprehensive text on the subject in 1969. Ptosis may be divided into congenital and acquired types.

Congenital ptosis is a developmental dystrophy of the levator muscle of unknown cause. The condition is usually sporadic, but it may be hereditary. Congenital ptosis may be simple, with a defect isolated to the levator muscle only or with superior rectus muscle weakness. Congenital ptosis also includes the blepharophimosis syndrome, which is hereditary and which, in addition to ptosis, may include varying degrees of telecanthus, epicanthus inversus, phimosis, and ectropion of the lower eyelids. Congenital ptosis also includes the Marcus Gunn jaw-winking syndrome, which is caused by an abnormal levator innervation between the mandibular division of the fifth cranial nerve and the third cranial nerve rather than a striated muscle fiber deficiency.

Acquired ptosis is best classified by Beard [1]; however, other authors such as Callahan, Frueh, and Rathbun [2] have added subclassifications. These include neurogenic, myogenic, aponeurotic, mechanical, traumatic, and pseudoptosis.

APONEUROTIC PTOSIS

Aponeurotic ptosis is thought to be the most frequent form of acquired ptosis. The condition may occur as the result of localized or generalized disinsertion or dehiscence of the aponeurosis from the tarsal plate. Clinical features of this type of ptosis may include a high or absent lid crease, good levator function, and thin eyelid tissues. Typically, aponeurotic ptosis occurs as a result of aging changes, including microinfarction of collagen bundles and other tissues within the aponeurosis [3]. Occasionally, levator fibers may be replaced with bundles of adipose tissue. This type of ptosis typically is found in older patients; however, younger patients may have aponeurotic ptosis as well. In addition to Rathbun's classification (Box 20-1), contact lens–induced ptosis is also common.

NEUROGENIC PTOSIS

Neurogenic ptosis may result from a multitude of neurologic disorders. This is most likely seen in third cranial nerve palsy, Horner's syndrome,

144 ORBITAL DISEASE

Box 20-1 Rathbun's Ptosis Classification

A. Aponeurotic Ptosis
1. Age
2. Blepharochalasis
3. Cataract or other ocular surgery
4. Chronic edema (Grave's disease, allergy)
5. Local blunt trauma

B. Myogenic Ptosis
1. Chronic progressive external ophthalmoplegia
2. Muscular dystrophy
3. Myasthenia gravis
4. Oculopharyngeal dystrophy
5. Trauma to the muscular levator

C. Neurogenic Ptosis
1. Horner's syndrome
2. Marcus Gunn jaw-winking ptosis
3. Misdirected oculomotor nerve palsy
4. Ophthalmoplegic migraine

D. Mechanical Ptosis
1. Excessive eyelid weight (eyelid or orbital mass)
2. Scarring

E. Pseudoptosis
1. Dermatochalasis
2. Globe malposition
3. Hypotropia
4. Lack of posterior eyelid support
5. Retraction of contralateral eyelid

ophthalmoplegic migraine, and multiple sclerosis. In third cranial nerve palsies, ptosis along with deficits of adduction, elevation, and depression of the eye may occur. The pupil may be normal or dilated. Lesions of the superior division of the third cranial nerve involve only the superior rectus and levator muscles with resultant ptosis and decreased levator function. Acquired third cranial nerve palsy may be a neurosurgical emergency if the pupil is involved, especially if the paralysis is due to a compressive lesion such as an aneurysm. Other causes of third cranial nerve palsies include infection, cavernous sinus thrombosis or fistula, tumors, contiguous paranasal sinus disease, and microinfarction of the nerve or midbrain.

Horner's syndrome consists of mild ptosis, pupillary miosis, upside-down lower lid ptosis, and at times, facial anhidrosis caused by decreased sympathetic tone to Müeller's muscle. Horner's syndrome is caused by a lesion somewhere in the sympathetic chain from the hypothalamus to the iris.

Ophthalmoplegic migraine is a rare cause of third cranial nerve palsy. Patients are typically young adults or children, often with a history of migraine headaches. Fifty percent of these patients have a family history of migraines. The mechanism of ophthalmoplegic migraine is unclear; however, it is believed that dilatation of the carotid artery may play a factor. Compression of the third cranial nerve usually occurs as the patient begins to complain of severe headaches, followed by ptosis and extraocular muscle paresis. The pupil is involved in the majority of patients. Magnetic resonance imaging (MRI) characteristically shows a thickened, enhanced nerve as it exits from the midbrain into the subarachnoid space [4].

MYOGENIC PTOSIS

Myogenic ptosis may sometimes overlap with ptosis of neurogenic or aponeurotic etiology. This includes myasthenia gravis, chronic progressive external ophthalmoplegia, and myotonic dystrophy. Myasthenia gravis is an autoimmune disease in which antibodies to acetylcholine receptors at the neuromuscular junction impair muscular contraction. In this situation, muscle fatigue and weakness occur. Myasthenia gravis is more common in women, although it affects all races and both genders. Approximately 85-90% of patients with myasthenia gravis present with localized ocular signs, although the disease may be generalized. Ptosis is the most frequent unilateral manifestation but may be unilateral or bilateral in nature. It usually worsens as the day progresses or with significant fatigue.

Chronic progressive external ophthalmoplegia is a disorder caused by a defect in the mitochondrial function in which a slowly progressive weakness of the extraocular and periocular muscles occurs. It is mostly autosomal dominant inheritance, although sporadic cases may occur. Chronic progressive external ophthalmoplegia involves the extraocular and periocular muscles, such as the orbicularis oculi. The iris and ciliary body muscles are not involved. It typically begins in childhood or adolescence and progresses very slowly over the next 40 to 50 years. Bilateral ptosis is usually the first symptom noted and subsequently any of the other body's muscles may be affected. At an advanced stage, the eyes may be totally immobile. Kerns and Sayre described a form of chronic progressive external ophthalmoplegia in which retinitis pigmentosa and complete heart block occur. Red, ragged fibers in muscle biopsies are suggestive of mitochondrial disease, as is the presence of spongy degeneration of the central nervous system. Patients with Kerns–Sayre syndrome require serial electrocardiograms to monitor for heart block.

Oculopharyngeal dystrophy is a myopathic dystrophy that begins after age 40 and consists of slowly progressive ptosis with dysphagia and dysarthria. This results from pharyngeal dystrophy and in some patients, the extraocular muscles; shoulder muscles and pelvic girdle muscles may be involved. Inheritance is autosomal dominant and may have a French-Canadian ancestry.

Myotonic dystrophy is a genetic disease with an autosomal dominant inheritance and may be associated with varying degrees of bilateral ptosis, orbicularis weakness or lid closure, extraocular muscle dysfunction, poor blinking, and dry eyes. Additional findings may include chromatic cataracts, testicular atrophy, frontal baldness, and first-degree heart block.

TRAUMATIC PTOSIS

Traumatic ptosis may occur from blunt or sharp trauma to the levator muscle or aponeurosis. Blunt or sharp injury may cause local damage to the levator muscle or aponeurosis, or both. Injury to the periocular tissues may cause edema, hemorrhage, or infection, which may also cause ptosis. Orbital fractures and foreign bodies may impair levator function either directly or indirectly. Ptosis may be shown to occur from injury to the levator aponeurosis as a result of ocular surgery, including cataract and trabeculectomy surgery, in up to 10-20% of cases. Contact lens–induced ptosis may occur in hard lens wearers who remove their contacts by stretching the eyelid with finger manipulation; from giant papillary conjunctivitis; or from a hard lens buried subconjunctivally.

MECHANICAL PTOSIS

Eyelid tumors, scarring, or blepharochalasis may cause mechanical ptosis. Lid tumors may cause ptosis as the result of increased weight on the upper lid or cause disinsertion by stretching the levator muscle. Cicatricial ptosis may be caused as a result of trauma or tumors.

PSEUDOPTOSIS

Pseudoptosis may appear with apparent ptosis when true eyelid ptosis is not actually present. This may be seen in lack of posterior lid support, such as in an anophthalmic eye or post-traumatic eye, or in the presence of an orbital prosthesis, which may result in ptosis. A hypotropic eye may appear to have a droopy eyelid, although this normalizes when the patient is asked fix on an object with the hypotropic eye. Dermatochalasis may also cause the appearance of a ptotic eyelid, although when lifting the skin off the eyelid, the margin typically returns to a normal position.

EVALUATION OF PTOSIS
History

It is important to determine whether the condition is congenital. In children, this is generally not a difficult task as parents who bring children for care usually know if the child was born with a ptosis or if a birth trauma caused it. Older patients with ptosis aren't sure of the time of its onset. Baby and childhood pictures are helpful in determining at what stage of life the patient had the ptosis [5].

A family history of ptosis is important.

A history of change is important. Is the condition improving, worsening, or has it remained stationary? Eyelid or globe surgery, as well as use of contact lenses, is also relevant.

Physical Examination

The examination of a patient with ptosis is probably the single most important factor in determining the type of surgical approach. Careful inspection and palpation of the eyelids and orbits helps determine the extent of asymmetry and proptosis, if present. In addition, palpation of the eyelids and orbital rims may detect orbital masses causing a mechanical ptosis on the lids. Everting the upper eyelid may also determine subconjunctival masses. Exophthalmometry may be helpful to assess for globe position and possible presence of orbital masses or enophthalmos. The position of the eyebrows, as well as head position, should be noted because the presence of ptosis may cause a compensatory posterior head posture.

Levator Function
By definition, levator function is the distance that the eyelid moves in millimeters from a maximum down-gaze to a maximum up-gaze without the eyebrow elevated. It is the single most important factor in the correct choice of surgical procedure. Levator function may be classified as excellent (13-15 mm), very good (10-13 mm), good (8-10 mm), fair (5-7 mm), and poor (4 mm or less).

The Amount of Ptosis
In unilateral ptosis, the amount of ptosis is measured as the distance between the upper and lower eyelid margins with the brow held in a relaxed position. The difference represents the amount of ptosis. The lower lid must be in normal position. In bilateral ptosis, the amount of ptosis is determined by the marginal reflex distance (MRD), that is, the light reflex from the cornea to the upper lid. The normal MRD is +4 to +4.5 mm with a normal eyelid position being 2 mm-1.5 mm below the superior limbus. Ptosis is classified as mild (2 mm), moderate (3 mm), and severe (4 mm). Check for ptosis in down-gaze [6]. The fissure in down-gaze is an indication of the ability of the levator muscle to relax. In congenital ptosis, the upper lid will lag behind the normal lid. In acquired ptosis, the lid is at a lower level than the normal lid.

Prominence of Lid Fold
This is a strong indicator of the degree of levator function.

Position of the Lid Fold
Accurate comparison of normal and abnormal lid folds must be determined so that the abnormal lid fold can be matched to the normal lid at surgery.

Lash Position
In severe ptosis, lash ptosis is also frequently present and can be improved at surgery.

The Amount of Upper Lid Skin
Excess upper lid skin will frequently be present in patients undergoing large levator resection or adult patients having ptosis correction. If this is suspected, a blepharoplasty along with ptosis surgery is appropriate.

Associated Lid Anomalies
Many syndromes such as blepharophimosis will have associated lid anomalies, which may be corrected by surgery at the same time the ptosis is corrected or at a later date.

Synkinetic Lid Movement
A classic example of this movement is Marcus Gunn jaw-winking ptosis, which represents abnormal congenital interconnections between the trigeminal nerve and the oculomotor nerve. In the resting state, the eyelid is ptotic. The eyelid elevates in response to movement of the external pterygoid muscle more commonly than to movements of the internal pterygoid muscle. The eyelid becomes more ptotic when the mandible is moved to the same side as the ptosis, and the eyelid retracts when the mandible moves to the opposite side, as during sucking or chewing. Other abnormal innervations must be considered such as aberrant regeneration of the third cranial (upper lid retraction on depression or adduction) and seventh cranial nerves.

Visual Acuity
Visual acuity must be tested because a significant number of children with ptosis will have amblyopia secondary to anisometropia and esotropia.

Fusion
A rapid Worth four-dot test or Titmus stereofly screening examination confirms normal function.

Extraocular Muscle Evaluation
Many patients with ptosis will have associated extraocular muscle imbalances or limitations, such as patients with chronic external ophthalmoplegia, myotonic dystrophy, or myasthenia gravis. Significant limitation of extraocular motility along with fair orbicularis tone will influence the final amount of levator surgery to avoid lid lag, lagophthalmos, and exposure keratopathy.

Bell's Phenomenon
This is a possible prognostic indicator of possible exposure problems if it is absent.

Tear Production
A Schirmer test is important in all adult-acquired ptosis to avoid complications of dry eye syndrome. A basic secretion test with topical anesthetic followed by a Schirmer strip in the inferior cul-de-sac for 5 minutes will determine basic secretion. Ten millimeters or more of moisture should be present on the filter paper strip. In addition, evaluation of tear film breakup time is also helpful (normal greater than 15 seconds).

Corneal Sensation
This test is usually not indicated unless a neurologic cause is suspected or a history of herpes simplex or Zoster is obtained.

Pupillary Signs

Rarely of diagnostic help except in Horner's syndrome and aberrant regeneration of the third cranial nerve.

Drug Testing

Tensilon Test

This test is indicated in all patients when myasthenia gravis is suspected. The test is done by giving 2 mg (0.2 cc) IV as a test dose to ensure the patient does not have a reaction, followed 30 seconds later by 8 mg (0.8 cc) and observing the patient's lid position. If the patient has myasthenia gravis, there will be a significant elevation in lid position within 1 to 5 minutes after giving the test dose. Cholinergic reactions are infrequent, but injectable atropine must be available as an antidote.

Cocaine and Hydroxyamphetamine Hydrobromide Solution (Paredrine)

This test is indicated in Horner's syndrome, which can occur from damage to any portion of the three-neuron oculosympathetic pathway. Maloney and colleagues reported the Mayo Clinic experience of 450 patients [7]. They were able to determine the etiology in 60% of these patients and found that 13% were central in origin, 44% were preganglionic, and 43% were postganglionic. It is important to determine whether a Horner's syndrome is central, preganglionic, or postganglionic because the nature of potential severity of the causative lesion varies considerably with the location. The lesions that cause completely isolated postganglionic Horner's syndrome are usually benign, whereas there is a high incidence of neoplasms and other serious disorders with isolated central and preganglionic Horner's syndrome. The pharmacologic tests require a two-step approach [8]. In the first step, two drops of solution of 10% cocaine are placed in the lower cul-de-sac of both eyes (the normal eye acts as a control) on two occasions 5 minutes apart. The eyes are examined every 15 minutes for the next 45 minutes. Cocaine blocks norepinephrine re-uptake by the nerve endings within the iris. Normal pupils dilate because of the persistent release and gradual accumulation of the neurotransmitter. Patients with a lesion of the sympathetic pathway in any of the three neurons show minimal or no pupillary dilatation because the amount of norepinephrine being released at the neurotransmitter junction of the iris is too small to produce dilatation. The Paredrine second step test separates the preganglionic and central portion of the system from the postganglionic portion. On a separate day, 1% hydroxyamphetamine hydrobromide solution is applied to both eyes in the same manner as was the cocaine. Paredrine directly causes the release of norepinephrine from the postganglionic nerve terminals. It will result in the dilatation of normal pupils and most miotic pupils from central and preganglionic lesions since the intact postganglionic neuron has stores of norepinephrine for release. However, postganglionic sympathetic neuron lesions result in eventual disappearance of the norepinephrine and no dilatation will occur during this test.

Neo-Synephrine Test

This test should be considered with all adult patients with acquired ptosis. This will help determine if, in fact, a unilateral ptosis is a bilateral ptosis based on Hering's law. Either 2.5% or 10% Neo-Synephrine may be used and is instilled into the cul-de-sac of the abnormal eye. If the ptotic lid rises at least 2 to 3 mm within 5 minutes, and the normal lid falls as compensation, bilateral ptosis is confirmed and, in addition, the patient may also be a candidate for a tarsal-conjunctival resection procedure or a conjunctival-Mueller's muscle resection surgery.

Other Tests

The ice test for myasthenia gravis [9,10]: application of a cold pack to the ptotic eye for 5 minutes that results in a marked improvement in the ptosis is suggestive of myasthenia gravis. This should be taken into consideration along with a variable ptosis, intermittent diplopia, positive fatigue test result, positive Cogan eyelid twitch test result, weakness of the orbicularis oculi, positive Tensilon test result, acetylcholine receptor antibodies, and an abnormal electromyograph test result. The possible explanation for the ice test may be equivalent to rest in short duration in testing or may affect the neuromuscular junction both by decreasing cholinesterase activity and by promoting efficiency of the acetylcholine and eliciting depolarization at the end plate.

TREATMENT

The various treatment modalities for congenital and acquired ptosis are beyond the scope of this chapter. In general, in congenital ptosis in its pure form, levator aponeurectomy or myectomy is indicated when levator function is fair to excellent. When levator function is below 5 mm, a frontalis sling is most appropriate. In acquired ptosis with good to excellent levator function and a good response to Neo-Synephrine, a Fasanella-Servat tarsal conjunctival Mueller's muscle resection or a Putterman conjunctival Mueller's muscle resection may be effective along with a levator aponeurosis advancement as the three choices. For anything less than good function, a levator aponeurosis advancement or myectomy is most appropriate. Finally, neuromuscular ptosis with poor levator function may be best managed with a frontalis sling.

PHOTOGRAPHY

Photographs should be taken of each patient preoperatively for preoperative planning, medicolegal reasons, and for insurance purposes.

CONSULTATION

The cause of acquired ptosis can sometimes be extremely difficult to determine. Therefore, interaction with an internist, endocrinologist, neurologist, or neurosurgeon may be helpful.

REFERENCES

1. Beard C. Ptosis. St. Louis: Mosby, 1969.
2. Harrington JN. Acquired blepharoptosis. In Stephenson CM (ed), Ophthalmic Plastic, Reconstructive and Orbital Surgery. Boston: Butterworth-Heinemann; 1997;138.
3. Dortzbach RK, Sutula FC. Involutional blepharoptosis: A histopathologic study. Arch Ophthalmol 1998;98:2045.
4. Siddens JD, Nesi FA. Acquired ptosis: classification and evaluation. In Nesi FA, Lisman RD, Levine MR (eds), Smith's Ophthalmic Plastic and Reconstructive Surgery. St. Louis: Mosby, 1998;379.
5. Beard C. Examination and evaluation of the ptosis patient. In Nesi, FA, Lisman, RD, Levine MR (eds), Smith's Ophthalmic Plastic and Reconstructive Surgery. St. Louis: Mosby, 1998;339.
6. Dryden RM, Kahanic DA. Worsening of blepharoptosis in down gaze. Ophthal Plast Reconstr Surg 1992;2:126.
7. Maloney WF, Young BR, Moyer NJ. Evaluation of the causes and accuracy of pharmacologic location in Horner's syndrome. Am J Ophthalmol 1980;90:394.
8. Striph GG, Miller NR. Disorders of eyelid formation caused by systemic disease. In Bosni AK (ed). Ophthalmic Plastic and Reconstructive Surgery. Philadelphia: WB Saunders, 1996;78.
9. Kubis KC, Danesh-Meyer HV, Savino PJ, et al. The ice test versus the rest test in myasthenia gravis. Ophthalmology 2000;107(11):1995.
10. Movaghar M, Slavin M. Effect of local heat versus ice on blepharoptosis resulting from ocular myasthenia. Ophthalmology 2000;107(12):2209.

21

Malignant Eyelid Lesions

OVERVIEW AND ETIOLOGY

Cutaneous carcinoma is the most common malignancy in the United States. Six hundred thousand people in this country are treated annually for basal or squamous cell carcinoma of the skin. Basal cell carcinoma occurs approximately four times as frequently as squamous cell carcinoma and almost 20 times more often than malignant melanoma [1]. Approximately 5-9% of all skin cancers arise in the eyelid. The most common malignancies of the periocular region are basal cell, squamous cell, sebaceous cell, and malignant melanoma. Among immunosuppressed patients, Kaposi's sarcoma is being recognized with increasing frequency [2]. Sunlight exposure (ultraviolet) is now recognized as an important etiologic factor in the development of epithelial malignancies. It is prevalent in fair-skinned individuals and is cumulative as reflected in the increasing incidence of tumor with advancing age. Basal cell carcinoma may occur in younger patients who have xeroderma pigmentosa or basal cell nevus syndrome. Most patients with basal cell carcinoma are older than 50 years of age, but approximately 5-15% of basal cell carcinomas occur in patients who are between 20 to 40 years old. Basal cell carcinoma is rare among black individuals. Approximately 70% of these tumors occur in the lower eyelid, 20% in the medial canthus, 7% in the upper lid, and 3% in the lateral canthus.

EXAMINATION

Basal cell carcinoma of the eyelids has a variety of clinical presentations. These presentations are most often dependent on the histologic characteristics. The most common histologic types of basal cell carcinoma include nodular, nodular ulcerative, pigmented, cystic, superficial spreading, and morpheaform. Nodular basal cell carcinoma, the most common, presents as a firm, pearly, dome-shaped nodule with telangiectatic vessels. The overlying epithelial surface appears smooth in appearance. The tumor is generally painless. Lesions may bleed spontaneously after minimal trauma. Other times, a tumor may outgrow its blood supply and develop a central ulceration with a crater with raised pearly borders leading to a common nodular ulcerative variant. The nodular type of tumor is the least aggressive and rarely has subcutaneous extensions, which are not clinically apparent, if present. Pigmented basal cell carcinoma is infrequent and is occasionally misdiagnosed as pigmented nevi or malignant melanoma. Cystic basal cell carcinoma may develop with mucin accumulation or degenerative necrosis within the solid tumor. Such carcinomas may be hard to distinguish from epithelial inclusion cysts or apocrine hidrocystoma. Morpheaform basal cell carcinoma appears as a flat, indurated plaque with telangiectasis. If situated along the lid margin, it may simulate a localized blepharitis, but with loss of lashes and distortion of lid margin architecture. The borders of morpheaform basal cell carcinoma may be indistinct with widespread subcutaneous involvement that is not visible clinically. After incomplete resection, the morpheaform type is ten times more likely to recur than the nodular type. Superficial spreading (multicentric) carcinoma is the least common and appears as erythematous, scaly patches with defined pearly borders and can be mistaken for eczematoid dermatitis or Bowen's disease [3].

TREATMENT

Suspicious eyelid lesions should be biopsied to establish a definitive diagnosis before complete excision and repair. Several treatment modalities have been used in the management of eyelid basal cell carcinomas. These include surgical excision, Mohs micrographic surgery, and radiation therapy. All have reported to achieve a 5-year cure rate of 90% or greater. Surgical excision with microscopic evaluation of the margins is the best technique for eliminating basal cell carcinoma. Frozen section control with tumor margins is performed by noting the clinical boundaries of the tumor edges and excising an additional 3-mm margin of normal-appearing tissue. If each of the margins examined by the pathologist is free of tumor, repair is undertaken. Surgical excision with frozen section control or Mohs micrographic surgery are the best treatment modalities with a 5-year cure rate of 95% or greater. Treatment cure is dependent on several variables, including location, size, and histologic characteristics of the basal cell carcinoma, immune status of the patient, and previous treatment failure. Basal cell carcinoma located in the medial canthus is more prone to be deeply infiltrative. Incompletely excised nodular basal cell carcinomas have been found to recur in 8% of cases, whereas ulcerative and morpheaform basal cell carcinomas have recurrence rates of 60% and 75%, respectively. Recurrent lesions have a propensity to be more aggressive and have a higher recurrence rate than primary tumors. Previously radiated tumors recur at a higher rate than lesions treated by other means. The majority of recurrent basal cell carcinoma occurs within 5 years of primary excision. Metastasis from a basal cell carcinoma is rare and these are generally lesions that are recurrent and extensive [4].

Squamous Cell Carcinoma

Overview and Etiology

Squamous cell carcinoma occurs less frequently than basal cell carcinoma, but it is a more aggressive and complicated tumor. Squamous cell carcinoma arises from differentiated cells of the epidermis that show maturation toward keratin formation, in contrast to basal cell carci-noma, which arises from the less well-differentiated basal cell layer. The average age of patients with squamous cell carcinoma is 70 years old. It typically occurs in patients with fair complexion who have a history of ultraviolet exposure. Patients with xeroderma pigmentosa and albinism have an increased incidence of squamous cell carcinoma at a young age. Patients with lymphoma, leukemia, and patients with immunosup-pression from organ transplantation have increased risk for squamous cell carcinoma.

Examination
Squamous cell carcinoma has a predilection for the lower eyelid. The classic type of lesion is an indurated, scaly, elevated plaque with a punched-out ulcerated area. The clinical appearance may vary from an ulcerated infiltrating mass to a verrucous elevated fungating nodular tumor. The tumor very frequently has a surface crusting because of the tendency of these anaplastic cells to form keratin. Most important, squamous cell carcinoma may be found at the base of a cutaneous horn and, therefore, it is important to biopsy the base of these lesions. The tumor is locally invasive; however, it can invade the orbit and sinus by continuous extension. Squamous cell carcinoma can also spread by a perineural invasion and lymphatic spread and metastasis to preauricular and submandibular lymph nodes in distant sites.

Patients with a diagnosis of atypical trigeminal neuralgia or painful ophthalmoplegia should be historically evaluated for past removal of a squamous cell skin carcinoma in the fifth cranial nerve distribution [5]. Actinic keratosis is considered a premalignant precursor to squamous cell carcinoma [6].

Treatment
Biopsy of the suspicious lesion is always performed before definitive surgical treatment. It is important to obtain representative deep sections of the tumor. Shave biopsies may miss dermal invasion or key factors in separating the benign lesions from the malignant lesions. Wide surgical excision with frozen section control of tumor margins is performed by noting the clinical boundaries of the tumor edge and excising an additional 5-mm cuff of normal-appearing tissue. The pathologist examines additional margins and, if free of tumor, immediate repair is undertaken.

Sebaceous Cell Carcinoma
Overview and Etiology
Sebaceous cell carcinoma is the third most common eyelid malignancy affecting middle-aged to older females more than males. Sebaceous cell carcinoma has a predilection for the upper lid over the lower lid due in part to the greater number of meibomian glands found in the upper eyelid. The upper and lower lids are simultaneously involved in approximately 10% of cases. Sebaceous cell carcinoma of the eyelids arises

most often in the meibomian glands in the tarsal plate, less often in the Zeis sebaceous glands of the lashes and, less frequently, in the caruncle and eyebrows [7]. These tumors can spread in an intraepithelial pagetoid fashion, which can involve the bulbar and palpebral conjunctiva. Less frequently, they can masquerade as conjunctivitis, blepharoconjunctivitis, or recurrent chalazia. Unlike basal cell carcinoma, squamous cell carcinoma and malignant melanoma, which have been linked to ultraviolet radiation. Unsaturated fatty acids (oleic acid) and radiation treatment have been associated with the development of sebaceous cell carcinoma. Sebaceous cell carcinoma can be classified with a degree of differentiation ranging from well differentiated to poorly differentiated lesions. There is an inverse relationship between the degree of sebaceous differentiation and mortality. Rao and coworkers found a 7% mortality rate for well-differentiated tumors and a 60% mortality rate for poorly differentiated tumors [8]. Other prognostic indicators include location of the tumor in the upper lid with delayed recognition over tumors of the lower lid, symptoms for longer than 6 months, an infiltrative growth pattern, moderate-to-poor sebaceous differentiation, and lymph node involvement.

Examination

The typical presentation of sebaceous cell carcinoma is a painless nodule believed to be a recurrent chalazion involving the upper eyelid. It may also present as a thickened eyelid margin or tarsal plate with a yellowish hue with associated lash loss or inflammation [9]. Ulceration of the lid margin is late compared with basal cell carcinoma or squamous cell carcinoma. Any patient with a chronic eyelid inflammation or recurrent chalazion that does not respond to medical or surgical treatment should have a generous, full-thickness eyelid biopsy. If sebaceous carcinoma is suspected, the pathologist should be made aware so the specimen can be stained with oil red O stain for fat.

Treatment

Surgical excision with microscopic frozen section evaluation of the margins and conjunctival mapping for pagetoid spread (intraepithelial spread) is the best technique for eliminating sebaceous carcinoma. A 5-mm cuff of normal appearing tissue from the clinical boundaries of the tumor edge is adequate. If no tumor cells are noted, immediate reconstruction is undertaken. Diffuse involvement of both upper and lower eyelids may necessitate exenteration [10]. Areas of concern include pagetoid spread to the bulbar conjunctiva, which may be treated with local conjunctival resection and cryotherapy. Preauricular or anterior cervical adenopathy may be treated with radical neck dissection or radiation therapy. The tumor is sensitive to radiation; however, radiation therapy is considered palliative and not curative. Sebaceous cell carcinomas recur in approximately 9-36% of patients. They may recur with orbital involvement in 6-17% of patients. Regional lymph nodes are the most common site of metastasis. Distant metastases include lung, liver, skull, and brain. The incidence of metastasis is approximately 17-28%. The 5-year mortality rate is approximately 30-40%.

Malignant Melanoma

Overview and Etiology

Malignant melanomas represent 5% of cutaneous cancers and less than 1% of malignant lesions of the eyelid. Melanomas may develop de novo, from preexisting nevi, or from lentigo maligna. The high-risk groups for melanoma are those with familial inheritance, patients with dysplastic nevus, and patients with high numbers of moles. The increased risk groups are patients with xeroderma pigmentosa, patients who have had multiple psoralen–ultraviolet A treatments, patients with cutaneous T-cell lymphoma, non-Hodgkin's lymphoma, and patients with organ transplants and acquired immunodeficiency syndrome. As for basal cell carcinoma and squamous cell carcinoma, melanomas are related to chronic ultraviolet radiation exposure. The principal types of cutaneous melanomas involving the eyelid are lentigo maligna melanoma and nodular melanoma, both of which are more common than superficial spreading melanoma. Lentigo maligna (Hutchinson's freckle) is the premalignant form of lentigo maligna melanoma. It is, in fact, malignant melanoma in situ. Lentigo maligna is most commonly noted on the face and eyelids. Lentigo maligna melanoma constitutes 90% of head and neck melanomas. All malignant melanomas arise from initial proliferation of atypical melanocytes within the epidermis. This phase of the disease is called the radial intraepidermal growth phase and may last for years. This is characteristic of lentigo maligna melanoma and superficial spreading melanoma. The vertical growth phase characteristic of nodular melanoma gives access to lymphatics and vasculature, which is associated with metastasis. Melanoma staging incorporates Clark's level of invasion and Breslow's thickness. Clark and coworkers developed a five-level classification based on anatomic landmarks but differentiation in the depth of dermal levels. The Breslow measurement of tumor thickness and the presence or absence of histologic ulceration is now considered to have more prognostic value in staging than the Clark classification [11,12]. It is a better prognostic indicator of 5- and 10-year survival. A melanoma of 0.76 mm thick or less will carry a 100% 5-year survival rate, whereas a melanoma of greater than 1.5 mm thick is associated with a 50-60% 5-year survival rate.

Examination

Lentigo maligna is the premalignant form of lentigo malignant melanoma, and appears as a nonpalpable, flat, tan-to-brown lesion with irregular margins. When the intraepithelial melanocytes invade the dermis, the area becomes elevated and darker and the melanoma form develops. The characteristic of superficial spreading melanoma is a flat-to-elevated lesion with irregular or notched edges and variegated colors of red, white, and blue. Nodular melanoma appears as a dark brown-to-black lesion.

Treatment

A complete excisional biopsy should be performed on all pigmented eyelid lesions suspected of being melanomas to determine the most appropriate staging. If the biopsy is positive for melanoma, metastatic workup is performed as these tumors metastasize to the lymph nodes, liver, lung, and other organ systems. If the metastatic workup results are negative, the melanoma is removed under frozen section control with a 0.5-cm margin for in situ melanoma, 1-cm margin for tumor thickness of less than 2 mm, and a 2-cm margin for tumor thickness greater than 2 mm according to the American Joint Committee on Cancer [13]. If these margins are negative, reconstruction is undertaken. Most recently, sentinel node biopsy and lymph node mapping have become the standard of care for staging of medium thickness malignant melanomas with a propensity for regional lymph node metastasis. Although the occurrence of malignant melanoma in the eyelid is uncommon and numbers of sentinel lymph node cases small, the technique may prevent unnecessary radical neck dissection. Adjuvant therapy, such as radiation, interferon, chemotherapy, or melanoma antibody therapy, is another consideration.

REFERENCES

1. Rodriguez-Sains, RS, Jakobiec FA. Eyelid and conjunctival neoplasm. In Nesi FA, Lisman RD, Levine MR (eds), Smith's Ophthalmic Plastic and Reconstructive Surgery (2nd ed). Philadelphia: Mosby, 1998;559.
2. Shields CL. Basal cell carcinoma of the eyelids. Int Ophthalmol Clin 1993;33:1.
3. Doxanas MT. Malignant epithelial eyelid tumors. In Bosniak (ed), Ophthalmic Plastic and Reconstructive Surgery. Philadelphia: WB Saunders, 1996;342.
4. Davies R, Briggs JH, Levine MR, et al. Metastatic basal cell carcinoma of the eyelid. Arch Ophthalmol 1995;113:634.
5. Miller NR, Newman NJ. Basal and squamous carcinoma of the skin. In Miller NR, Newman NJ (eds), Walsh and Hoyt's Clinical Neuro-ophthalmology (Vol. 2), (5th ed). Philadelphia: Williams & Wilkins 1998;2457.
6. Reifler DM, Hornblass A. Squamous cell carcinoma of the eyelids. Surg Ophthalmol 1986;30:349.
7. Rodriguez-Sains, RS, Jakobiec FA. Eyelid and conjunctival neoplasm. In Nesi FA, Lisman RD, Levine MR (eds), Smith's Ophthalmic Plastic and Reconstructive Surgery (2nd ed). Philadelphia: Mosby, 1998;559.
8. Rao NA. Sebaceous carcinoma of the ocular adnexa. Hum Pathol 1982;13:113.
9. DePotter P, Shields CL, Shields JA. Sebaceous gland carcinoma of the eyelid. Int Ophthalmol Clin 1993;33:5-9.
10. Reifler D. Eyelid tumors. In Stephenson (ed), Ophthalmic Plastic Reconstructive and Orbital Surgery. Boston: Butterworth-Heinemann, 1997;213.
11. Rodriguez-Sains RS, Jacobiec FA, Iwamoto T. Lentigo maligna of the lateral canthal skin. Ophthalmology 1981;88:1186.
12. Swetter SM, Ross MI. The rationale behind the 2002 AJCC Melanoma Staging Committee Recommendations. The Melanoma Letter, vol. 19, no. 4, 2001. New York: The Skin Cancer Foundation.
13. Li LJ. Surgical margins for malignant melanoma. Melanoma Update 2002 Symposium, University Hospitals of Cleveland, October 23, 2002.

22

Lacrimal Gland Tumors

OVERVIEW AND ETIOLOGY

The lacrimal gland can harbor a variety of types of tumors and inflammations, accounting for 5-13% of all orbital masses [1]. Although there are variations from series to series, previous reports have indicated that approximately 50% of lacrimal gland tumors are of epithelial origin and 50% are of nonepithelial origin. In the category of epithelial tumors, pleomorphic adenoma accounts for approximately 50% of the cases, adenoid cystic carcinoma 25%, and other primary carcinomas 25% (Box 22-1 and Table 22-1). Among the nonepithelial lesions 50% are lymphoid tumors and 50% are various forms of idiopathic orbital inflammation. It is important to appreciate, however, there are other, more recent series of cases that have a smaller percentage of epithelial tumors (Boxes 22-2 and 22-3).

Pleomorphic adenoma is a painless, slowly growing tumor of the lacrimal gland that occurs predominantly among middle-aged persons, occurring more commonly in women than in men. Malignant mixed tumors occur in a similar age range with equal gender distribution. The malignant component may be adenoid cystic carcinoma, adenocarcinoma, or squamous cell carcinoma. Adenoid cystic carcinomas are the primary epithelial malignancy of the lacrimal gland, occurring in either gender with a peak incidence around the fourth decade, but may present

Box 22-1 Lacrimal Gland Masses

50% are epithelial tumors
50% are benign
50% are malignant
50% are nonepithelial tumors

Table 22-1 Features of 190 Epithelial Tumors of Lacrimal Gland

Type	Cases	%
Mixed pleomorphic	127	67
Benign pleomorphic	102	54
Malignant	25	13
Carcinomas not related to mixed	63	33
Adenoid cystic	53	28
Adenocarcinoma	10	5

From Zimmerman, L., MD. Armed Forces Institute of Pathology — Yearly Conference, 1970.

Box 22-2 Lacrimal Gland Tumors	
120 Tumors	
Inflammatory	63%
Epithelial origin	34%
Malignant lymphoma	3%
Epithelial Tumors	
41 Tumors	
Benign mixed tumors	41%
Adenoid cystic carcinoma	29%
Adenocarcinoma	5%
Malignant mixed tumor	17%
Metastatic carcinoma	7%

From Font RL, Smith SL, Bryan RG. Malignant epithelial tumors of the lacrimal gland: a clinico-pathologic study of 21 cases. Arch Ophthalmol 1998;116:613.

rarely in childhood [2]. Histopathologic morphology shows the cribriform variant (Swiss cheese) to have a better prognosis than the basaloid pattern. Other histopathologic subtypes are sclerosing, comedo, and tubular [3]. Adenocarcinomas are much rarer, predominant in males, and present in an older age group than adenoid cystic carcinoma. Squamous cell carcinoma and mucoepidermoid carcinoma are extremely uncommon lacrimal gland tumors.

Pleomorphic adenomas are composed of proliferating ductal elements occurring in a myxoid or hyaline stroma with or without calcification. The slowly expanding tumor compresses the surrounding lacrimal tissue to form a pseudocapsule [4]. The orbital lobe of the lacrimal gland is most predominantly involved; though, less commonly, the palpebral lobe can be involved. Presentation of a lacrimal gland tumor, therefore, depends on where in the orbital lacrimal gland it starts to grow. If, for example, the tumor starts anteriorly or at the head of the lacrimal gland, a visible palpable mass may be seen with no diplopia or globe displacement. If the tumor starts in the body of the gland, fullness in the lacrimal fossa

BOX 22-3 Clinical Review of 142 Cases of Lacrimal Gland Lesions

78% of lacrimal gland lesions were of nonepithelial origin
22% were primary epithelial neoplasms

Nonepithelial lesion
Inflammation (64%)
Granulomatous
Nongranulomatous
Lymphoid tumor (14%)
Reactive lymphoid hyperplasia
Malignant lymphoma

Epithelial lesion
Dacryops (6%) (lacrimal gland cysts)
Pleomorphic adenoma (12%)
Malignant epithelial tumors (4%)

Source: Shields CL, Shields JA. Clinicopathologic review of 142 cases of lacrimal gland lesions. Ophthalmology 1989;96:431.

is seen but may not be palpable; however, the globe may be displaced inferior medially and diplopia may be present on elevation and abduction. Finally, if the tail or posterior aspect of the lacrimal gland is involved, no mass or fullness or diplopia is observed, but a significant amount of proptosis may be present. Palpebral lobe tumors present with a palpable mass underneath the lid with alteration of lid contour.

The natural course of the lacrimal gland tumor, especially the pleomorphic adenoma, is one of slow progression over approximately 6 months to several years before the patient sees a physician. Malignant transformation in a pleomorphic adenoma is evident by an acceleration of symptoms and signs. It has been estimated that up to 20% of pleomorphic adenomas may undergo malignant transformation within 30 years after inadequate surgical excision or biopsy.

Primary malignant lacrimal gland tumors have a much shorter history of duration of weeks to months. They tend to be infiltrating to periosteum and bone and can invade the temporalis fossa, cranial diploë, or intracranial space. Perineural invasion (lacrimal nerve) is very common in adenoid cystic carcinoma and accounts for much of its spread and extension. Pain is a prominent feature. Lacrimal gland lymphoma is present in approximately 24% of patients at the time of presentation and develops late in another 9%. Orbital pain is rare with lacrimal gland lymphoma.

CLINICAL FEATURES

The clinical features of pleomorphic adenoma of the lacrimal gland are a slowly progressive (6 months to 1 year), firm, relatively painless mass in superior temporal orbit. Proptosis, globe displacement, diplopia, fullness, or a palpable mass may or may not be present. In contrast, a malignant lacrimal gland tumor may have a short course of weeks to a few months with proptosis, globe displacement, diplopia, and pain from perineural invasion.

INVESTIGATION

High-resolution computed tomography (CT) scans for pleomorphic adenoma show a well-circumscribed, round-to-oval mass of heterogeneous density in the lacrimal gland fossa with or without globe displacement [5]. There may be no bone involvement or saucerization of bone secondary to a pressure effect. Conversely, rapidly growing or soft tissue tumors, such as primary carcinoma or lymphoma, are less well defined, irregular and poorly demarcated, and mold to the contour of the globe. The primary carcinomas frequently extend along the lateral orbital wall, displacing the lateral rectus extending toward superior orbital fissure or track retrograde along the lacrimal nerve. Calcification occurs as diffuse flecks in approximately one third of the lacrimal gland carcinomas and is relatively rare in pleomorphic adenomas. Magnetic resonance imaging (MRI) shows an irregular mass infiltrating along the lateral rectus. A T1-weighted image shows the mass hyperintense to muscle but hypointense to fat. Signals become hyperintense to orbital fat on T2-weighted images [6].

DIFFERENTIAL DIAGNOSIS

When symptoms have been present for more than 10 to 12 months in the absence of pain, the differential diagnosis is pleomorphic adenoma, lymphoma, sarcoidosis, and chronic dacryadenitis. On high-resolution CT scan, pleomorphic adenoma has a round or oval configuration, tends to flatten the globe and expand, but not destroy the bone of the lacrimal gland fossa. A lacrimal gland mass that molds to the globe is suggestive of lymphoma, chronic dacryadenitis, or sarcoidosis, with these diagnoses being more likely if the mass is bilateral. Conversely, a rapidly expanding, ill-defined, painful mass with bony destruction on CT scan is suggestive of malignant lacrimal gland tumor. Finally, an acute onset of a painful swollen and tender lacrimal gland is likely inflammatory or idiopathic orbital inflammation that should respond rapidly with system antibiotics or steroids [7].

PROGNOSIS AND TREATMENT

The prognosis for primary epithelial malignancy of the lacrimal gland is poor even with extensive surgery and radiation therapy. Survival rates are less than 50% at 5 years and 20% at 10 years. In Wright's series of 38 patients, only two survivors were disease-free after a follow-up period of 16 years [8]. Font and Gamel's series reported a survival rate of 20% at 10 years regardless of the treatment regimen. They document a recurrence rate of 55-80% within 5 to 6 years [9,10].

Pleomorphic adenomas should be excised intact with a cuff of normal tissue via lateral orbitotomy. Appropriate decision making with biopsy of the pleomorphic adenoma with spillage of the tumor cells may lead to recurrence and malignant transformation. Primary malignant lacrimal gland tumors are very problematic, leading to recurrence, perineural spread, intraorbital and intracranial extension, and widespread metastasis. A new multidisciplinary treatment protocol appears promising. It consists of preoperative cytoreductive intracarotid chemotherapy, postoperative intravenous chemotherapy, conventional orbital exenteration, and radiation therapy [6].

REFERENCES

1. Shields JA. Epithelial tumors of the lacrimal gland. In Shields JA (ed), Diagnosis and Management of Orbital Tumors. Philadelphia: WB Saunders, 1989.
2. Font RL, Gamel JS. Epithelial tumors of the lacrimal gland; an analysis of 265 cases. In Jakobiec FA (ed), Ocular and Adnexal Tumors. Birmingham, Alabama: Aesculapius, 1978.
3. Gamel JW, Font RL. Adenoid cystic carcinoma of the lacrimal gland: the clinical significance of a basaloid histologic pattern. Hum Pathol 1982;13:219.

4. Levine MR, Larson DW. Orbital tumors. In Pudus SM, Yanoff M (assoc. ed.), Tenzel RR, (eds), Textbook of Ophthalmology, (Vol. 4). New York: Gower Medical Publishers, 1993.

5. Jakobiec FA, Yeo JH, Trukel SL, et al. Combined clinical and computer tomographic diagnosis of primary lacrimal fossa lesions. Am J Ophthalmol 1982;94:785.

6. Tse DT. A new treatment protocol for adenoid cystic carcinoma of the lacrimal gland. Presented at the 40th Anniversary Bascom Palmer Eye Institute Conference, Miami, Florida, February 2002: Bascom Palmer Eye Institute.

7. Rose GE. Lacrimal gland neoplasia. In Bosniak S (ed), Principles and Practice of Ophthalmic Plastic and Reconstructive Surgery, (Vol. 2). Philadelphia: WB Saunders, 1996;999.

8. Wright JE, Rose GE, Garner A. Primary malignant neoplasms of the lacrimal gland. Br J Ophthalmol 1992;76:401.

9. Font RL, Gamel JW. Adenoid cystic carcinoma of the lacrimal gland: a clinicopathologic study of 79 cases. In Nicholson DH (ed), Ocular Pathology Update. New York: Masson Publishing, 1980.

10. Font RL, Smith SL, Bryan RG. Malignant epithelial tumors of the lacrimal gland: a clinicopathologic study of 21 cases. Arch Ophthalmol 1998;116:613.

Index

---

www.ingramcontent.com/pod-product-compliance
Lightning Source LLC
Chambersburg PA
CBHW070722220326
41598CB00024BA/3256